Traditional Healing:
New Science or New Colonialism?
(Essays in Critique of Medical Anthropology)

Edited with an Introduction by

Philip Singer, Ph.D.

Allport College of Behavioral Sciences
Oakland University, Rochester, Michigan

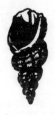

CONCH MAGAZINE LIMITED (PUBLISHERS)
Owerri   New York   London
1977

First published 1977

Printed in the United States of America

Library of Congress Catalog Card Number
75-18490

ISBN: 0-914970-36-4

Library of Congress Cataloging in Publication Data

CONTENTS

INTRODUCTION:
FROM ANTHROPOLOGY AND MEDICINE TO "THERAPY" AND NEO-COLONIALISM

Philip Singer, Ph.D.

Of the contributors to this volume, Snow, Messing and Singer are social scientists-anthropologists. Araneta, Ruiz, Westermeyer are psychiatrists-practitioners; Williams is a general practitioner, now in a psychiatric residency; Lambo and Mume are traditional healers; as a candidate for the doctorate in Public Health, Mburu is a practitioner-change-agent; Dawkins is a revolutionary; Shepherd is an attorney; and Langrod a medical-social research scientist. Onyioha is an educated Nigerian who believes a synthesis is possible.

It was only when I began to classify the contributors by occupation that the insight came to me that Araneta, Ruiz and Westermeyer were *not* social scientists, but indeed practitioners. It came as a surprise because I think that for too long anthropologists, qua culture and personality social scientists, have been thinking of psychiatrists as social scientists. By virtue of their training, however, psychiatrists are first clinicians, and secondly scientists. Anthropologists are first and foremost by training social scientists, although a few, such as George Devereux, may become clinicians.

After an association of many years with psychiatrists in a variety of field and academic situations, I have come to the conclusion that what we have in common is our blinders to values and our reliance upon a so-called ethical neutrality. For the social scientist this appears under the rubric of objectivity in data gathering; for the psychiatrist it is justified as relief from symptoms of the suffering patient. The anthropologist, especially in the "medical anthropology" field, suffers from "empiricism," the psychiatrist with pretension as social scientist, may be said to suffer from "clinicism."

In trying to put together this collection of articles around the theme of "Traditional Healing, New Science or New Colonialism?" I deliberately wanted to raise the question of the "correctness" of the "clinical" and "empirical" approaches in relation to the larger question of values and societies. Is relief of functional distress, anxiety verging on

1

panic, psychosomatic illness, psychotic acting out, etc., sufficient unto themselves without additionally raising the questions of significance, of the *meaning* of the symptomatic distressed behavior, the methods used to quell the behavior, and the nature of the society in which such cultural behavior takes place?

Much to my distress, I have observed over the years that anthropologists who enter the field of culture and personality or medical anthropology, tend to think they have performed their obligations as social scientists fully if they have learned to take a fuller "history" than their psychiatric colleagues, and put that history in a cultural context.

"Significance" for them then becomes the additional input they can provide the psychiatrist-clinician as the therapist tries to help the patient. However, "significance" in terms of values, better or worse, good or bad, right or wrong, is rarely raised. There is a parallel here with the way anthropologists worked under the colonial rule of the British, Dutch and French. Although there was descriptive, ethnographic work done, it was largely in the service of maintaining the structure of colonialism.[1] Although there is descriptive, medical anthropology work done, most of it seems to be in the service of therapy and anthropology as an academic discipline.

Let us take for example the medical anthropological, or clinical psychiatric, problem of jealousy.[2]

From the clinical psychiatric viewpoint, possessive jealousy and ideas of paranoid infidelity is a problem for the physician. The recommendation is made that therapy must be undertaken with both the man and woman involved. The approach recommended is one of rationally uncovering the sources of insecurity which lie behind the jealous individual. Openness, honesty and therapy on transactional lines is recommended.

Jealousy is also a problem to be encountered in Nigeria. How is it to be handled, for example, in Yoruba culture? Briefly, with magic and witchcraft and coercive rituals. For example: A man and woman have been having a sexual relationship for some years. The man becomes jealous, suspicious because the woman refuses to have sex with the frequency demanded by the man. The man goes to the traditional healer, who will provide the therapy of "punishment." The traditional healer has in his therapeutic armamentarium a ritual which will make it impossible for the woman to have sex with any man. Within a few months, the woman will "come begging." One of the techniques used by the jealous man on the allegedly unfaithful woman is to cause her to pass over a knotted string stretched over her path. The effect of the knots is to tighten the vagina so that no penis may enter. When the man wishes to "redeem" the woman, he need only untie the knots. It is believed that such women are "werewolves" who are not content with one man. Another way the wronged (jealous) man may get revenge is by causing the woman and her lover to become carnally "stuck together" and in that way to be brought to the hospital to the shame of both. As Chief Lambo says, in discussing these techniques, "There are wonders in nature."

These "wonders in nature" are part of the traditional cultural pattern of the people. But that does not, and should not, make them immune from criticism. Colonization of the Indirect Rule which both suppressed as "evil" the traditions of the people, creating the conditions for cultural genocide, and alienation, and which made free access to the progress of the Colonial master impossible, is not the issue. What is at issue is the new Colonialism of the independent countries which makes access to the progress of the urban rulers equally impossible for the masses and supports the traditions of the past as if they were things that are true and good, but only for the masses, not the rulers. For the hegemony of the white colonialists has been supplanted by the hegemony of the black rulers. Whether or not the African who employs the traditional healer is less alienated than the African who chooses to consult the Westernized marriage counselor is beside the point. The point is, which is preferable, and of course, what makes it so? Magic and superstition in a traditional cultural context, or a more rational approach to interpersonal problems of living? Traditionalism is as much a "force" and a "social process" as is colonialism. Because it is "traditional" does not make it "better" or anti-colonial.

What I am suggesting here is that the continued use,

3

and promotion of traditional healers is part of a continuing socio-economic exploitation, and needs to be looked at structurally as part of the failure of the newly independent countries and our own to develop a national system of health care for all. Although the educated African may indeed seek out the traditional healer, as Chief K.O.K. Onyioha demonstrates, he also has access to the Western materia medica as well, and uses it. The poor African does not. Dr. Snow's paper on "The Religious Component in Southern Folk Medicine" addresses the problem for the United States.

Just as the dominant colonial interests of the past influenced anthropologists, either with awareness, or out of awareness, to justify the prevailing system (Lewis, *ibid.*, p. 583); we have the same situation with anthropologists and psychiatrists today in relation to so-called problems of mental illness. I hasten to add here that it is the approach to mental illness as pathology, justifying the imposition of a special class of "healer," that is the cutting edge of this new colonialism, and that it doesn't make any difference whether the cultural drama is acted out in Nigeria, where Chief Lambo sees his patients, or the South Bronx, where Dr. Ruiz sees his, or Pontiac, Michigan, where Dr. Williams sees his. In this sense I am not emphasizing the *differences* between Western "civilized" culture and the other culture's (whatever it may be) "superstition," but rather the similarities in terms of differential treatment. The poor, the powerless, wherever they happen to be, are the natives of colonialism. To say, as many psychiatrists and mental health personnel do, that social stress is reflected in "psychological disorders" is a brand of reductionism which can only perpetrate exploitation by "medically" relieving so-called stress-pathology.

In this sense, the relationship between the individual and society, or culture and personality, can be looked at as one of continuing potential conflict and stress, usually between the haves and the have nots, the powerful and the less powerful. Responsibility for dealing with this conflict, typically lies with the political institutions of the state, which, of course, include the health system.

The entire concept of mental illness has developed in such a way as to encompass a wide range of what we may call "stressed" behaviors which declare the incapability, or unwillingness, of the individual(s) to adjust their actions to the conditions and rules of society currently in existence. Thus, arson in the South Bronx, where housing conditions are horrendous, would be considered and is so considered, grounds for considering whether or not the arsonist is mentally sick. Similarly, Soviet scientists who write outside of their area are committed to mental institutions because of their dissident view of their society. Thus, the "mental illness" model provides a cross-cultural base to explain a wide range of anti-social and "illegal" behaviours. "Therapy" then becomes the control device for the social system and a means for implementing a *political* concept of responsibility, or oppression. How convenient it is for so-called colonialists, and so-called anti-colonialists, to know that mental illness is no respector of ideology and there is probably just as much schizophrenia (whatever that may be) in one country as in the other. That way cultural relativity, and political oppression, are both preserved by *recognizing* the symptoms of schizophrenia with due attention to cultural "masking," and then applying "therapy," in the service of the state, whether colonialist, capitalistic, or communistic. From a traditional, relativistic, anthropological viewpoint, it is just as valid for the Soviet biologist Medvedev, or the intellectual Bukovsky to be committed to a mental hospital, as it is for a suicidal, alcoholic or drug addicted person in the West, to be "treated" via commitment to a mental institution, or by becoming addicted to an approved drug of choice, Methadone, instead of Heroin, in the United States. Yet, I seriously doubt whether there will be many, if any anthropologists who would defend the imprisonment of the Soviet dissident intellectuals, although they will defend the use of magic and superstition.

But if, as anthropologists and social scientists we can agree that the forms of functional mental illness may be defined only with respect to the cultural forms of behavior in that society, then we should also be prepared logically to accept the forms of political sanctions (therapy) as part of that same social context, and be just as tolerant of them. But obviously, we are not. Why not? I suggest that it is so because some values are more important to us than others, if

we happen to be Western social scientists. To confine someone in a geographically remote, occupational labor therapy
work setting, is somehow repulsive to our values, whereas to
pretend that a non-existent snake has been removed from
someone's belly, as described by Mume, is not. Any discussion of therapy for the mentally ill must be concerned
with the intermingling of political and therapeutic concepts,
or, as the anthropologist would put it, with culture and
personality, and how this affects and shapes political-legal-
clinical processes and institutions.

Oscar Lewis' "culture of poverty" may be somewhat in
academic disrepute as obvious theorizing that perpetuates
poverty and resists social change, but the awareness that the
"culture of mental illness" plays the same role, has not yet
been made with the exception of such pioneers as the
psychiatrist Thomas Szasz. Anthropologists in the "medical
anthropology" field, perhaps one of the fastest growing in the
discipline, also enjoy the possibility of being both "applied"
and "pure." Every time an anthropologist sees a patient
possessed, and then exorcized, or whatever the situation may
be, he is witnessing in a relatively short span of time an entire
process of social change, and he cannot but have the feeling
(as I have had) that just by being there, in the healing setting,
he has somehow participated in the process of therapy, of
"clinical" work. "Applied" anthropology may still have low
status, "clinical" anthropology does not. Indeed some
anthropologists apparently would like to substitute the
anthropologist for the Id.[3]

As a result of being the host in my home for Chief
Lambo for one month (February 1974) during which time he
delivered a series of lectures on "Traditional Healing" to
Oakland University, I found some of the issues I raise
here, to be sharply, indeed cruelly, raised in my everyday
problems of living with Chief Lambo and, indeed, they
continue even now while he is back in Lagos.

While he was here, the traditional role of the anthropologist became fuzzy, to say the least. As a result of publicity, which I materially assisted in arranging, on radio,
newspaper, and television, over 100 persons black and white,
young and old, male and female, educated and functionally

6

illiterate, made contact with me because they wanted help from Chief Lambo. They came with a variety of complaints, and all had been to the physician many times before. They came with sleeplessness, bad luck, a pet dog with diagnosed cancer of the jaw, alcoholism, barrenness, asthma, obesity, impotency, hexes, etc. As host, anthropologist, scientist, voyeur, professor (but not clinician), I was able to sit in on the sessions with each patient, and with the consent of all parties, to record the interaction. Chief Lambo diagnosed one and all on the basis of Rosicrucian medical astrology, his own Yoruba beliefs about witchcraft, and herbal remedies, which as his anthropological-host-apprentice, I helped prepare from his stock, on the kitchen stove. The examining procedure was simple. An initial fee was paid, the patient related what was bothering him, Chief Lambo then consulted his Rosicrucian medical astrology text, performed some Ifa calculations based on birthdate, prescribed a herbal remedy and accepted an additional fee. There was no suggestion of any empiricism in his approach, and to that extent it was completely a product of supernaturalism. *All* complaints were declared to be curable, "no problem." *None* of the persons who came, including some from Northern Michigan, raised any questions, any doubts, and all were prepared to pay whatever was asked.

This was no longer a question of watching the Kali Mai healer in Guyana, or the Zar healer in Ethiopia, or the Spiritualistas in the Bronx. This was in my home, and I thought I knew better. It seemed clear to me that what I was witnessing was exploitation of both functional and organic disorders. The functional might obtain symptomatic relief (a number did); some of the organic situations might go into spontaneous remission (none did to my knowledge); but what about my own values, my own convictions, my own sense of responsibility, that what I was participating in as anthropological host, was exploitation? If, in the field, I had no "right" to impose my values on my host culture, did I have the right to feel "responsible" as host to the representative of another culture?

To further complicate the situation, was the fact that there was a great deal of money potentially to be gained by joining with Chief Lambo, in providing herbs. "Perhaps I should open a herbal shop?" It was partly out of that consideration that I solicited the contribution from Shepherd. His major point is that whether or not something is legal (ethical) depends upon usage and norms and mores. Is that what anthropology was about? Was it, is it, a marketable commodity? To the extent that any anthropologist is paid, in the university, the terminal cancer ward, the museum, the applied research project, AID, War on Poverty, etc., he is certainly marketing his knowledge commodity. Well, what difference is opening up a shop with an "informant?" Was that what Chief Lambo was? Indeed, who was the informant and who was the anthropologist? To the extent that I was his host, I was his informant. To the extent that he used me to help understand the chief complaints of the persons who come to see him, I was his informant. After a time, I think I also became identifiable as a person and friend. As a partner in a herbal shop I would certainly learn a great deal. And after all, isn't *that* what anthropology is all about? The pursuit of knowledge?[4]

While groping for the right questions, and grappling with the implications of the questions I had raised, I found no comfort at all in the academic notion that the development of ethics is central to and part of the evolutionary[5] process. If there was indeed an ethical unity of mankind, in relation to these questions, I could not find it while introspecting my genes. Why, I wondered, was it possible for anthropologists, from an anthropological viewpoint of the psychic unity of mankind, to oppose any form of racism as both morally and scientifically indefensible, and to actively take a stand against Nazism, and yet not take a similar stand against all forms of colonialism, especially medical colonialism?

What was it about illness, mental illness in particular, and traditional healers, that could cause anthropologists to salute the flag of cultural relativity and "therapy," and cause such hesitancy about taking a stand as to one form of treatment (therapy) being better, or worse, than another?

Ruiz, Araneta, Williams, indeed all the contributors to this volume, have noted the fact that social problems contribute to mental illness. Indeed, the medical director of one community mental health center[6] in Philadelphia in the United States is on record as categorically stating that social factors may be the chief precipitating factor. Nevertheless, the heart of the Philadelphia training program for the non-professional (sic) Mental Health Assistants, most of whom are black, women, with less than a high school education, is "sensitivity training," or "becoming psychologically minded."[7] Their great asset, according to the psychiatrist who is the Director of the Crisis Center, is that "The mental health assistant bridges the culture gap. She understands the patients that we have."[8] Yet, despite the fact that the performance of these indigenous non-professionals is rated in relation to chronically psychotic people as better than the physicians, they start at $3,900 up to a maximum of $5,500. However, in the process of working in the Mental Health Center, there is a problem that causes the non-professional some bad marks, and perhaps contributes to low pay. That is the problem of "creeping professionalism," where some mental health assistants attempt to follow "traditional therapeutic practices."[9]

What an impossible bind for the professional to put the non-professional in. At the same time, it illustrates beautifully the enlightened psychiatric clinical approach, which has nothing to do with organic "clinical" baselines, but everything to do with normative propositions concealing value judgements.[10]

As Doctor Panzetta, Director of the Crisis Center and the Psychosocial Clinic in the Philadelphia ghettos is quoted as saying:

> Since the Center stresses flexibility of treatment and since it values the basic intuitive talents of the assistants, the tendency to set up rigid schedules and rely solely on 'word therapy' is discouraged.[11]

I would suggest that much of the confusion over values, ethics, judgements, particularly on the part of psychiatrists and anthropologists comes from the continuing confusion between functional and organic. This is a confusion which is supported by all the prestige of so-called "scientific" medicine in the United States, especially the major drug companies, which have a very heavy investment indeed in functional, behavioral manipulation through organic means. Thus, for example, a major drug company, Roche Laboratories, puts out a three-part cassette series for free distribution to physicians, with the title: "The Natural Processes of Healing," with a panel made up of an anthropologist, a biologist, a psychologist, a psychoanalyst and a physician. The emphasis on the tapes is the importance of the "social context" to the healing process, and the fact that we really know so little about the mind-body continuum, etc., etc. Each cassette contains both a verbal plug, and a handout on the value of Valium therapy which will help the patient, of course with the physician counseling "to understand that much of his tension and anxiety can be relieved by your reassurance and counseling, and that these measures can do more than any medicine to help him cope with his basic problems. The patient is reassured in knowing he can expect his medication, Valium, to help him avoid feeling overwhelmed by his symptoms."

However, as one of the Roche panelists, A. R. Feinstein, Professor of Medicine and Epidemiology, Yale University School of Medicine, cautions, when the other experts seem to be getting carried away with the "natural processes," one should not forget the good things that organic specialization and the organic concept of disease has led to in medicine. Among the good things is specialization, including such things as surgery, antibiotics, orthopedics, obstetrics/gynecology, etc. At the same time the Doctor acknowledges, as a good clinician, that he is prepared to accept any help he can get from any source, "whether it be the shaman, psychoanalyst, or the pharmaceutical substance."

This catholicity of the clinical approach is certainly to be welcomed in the developed West. However, the organic, scientific approach has hardly yet been made available to all who need it in the underdeveloped countries. To equate the clinical pragmatics of the West, with the magic and superstition of most traditional healers, is to further cause confusion in this already confused area of the functional and the organic. Yet that is precisely what the United States is doing, where all kinds of behavior become "psychosocial disturbances."[12] But surely, clinical pragmatics can hardly be equated with psychotherapeutic gnosis which would submerge all kinds of behavior, including the rage of the exploited. Dawkins, in his paper, has caught that rage well, and points up the fact that the normative implicit values in psychiatry gain currency only because of the camouflage of the "medical model."

This "medical model" has become so all absorptive, all pervasive, that it bears the possibility of accommodating all deviance, all outrage, all "non-adaptive" behavior. By now it is commonplace to hear that from 50-80 percent of the problems brought before the general practitioner are psychosomatic, or functional in origin. Dr. Count Gibson, chairman of the Department of Family, Community and Preventive Medicine at the Stanford University School of Medicine, is quoted as saying that the training of the internists is hospital based and focused on the diseases, and not the person. He adds that a half of the problems encountered in primary care are emotional. At least the religious model is prepared to admit that some things are secular, but not the medical-psychiatric-cultural model. Indeed, the medical model combined with the cultural model is one of the most important vectors for the continuing exploitation of peoples. Invariably one talks or writes about the importance of the "cultural broker," whether that be in the South Bronx, or Philadelphia, or Mexico, by which they mean the non-professional. The interesting thing is that the emphasis on the cultural broker will be made regardless of data which indicates that they are not necessary. For example, the anthropologist Rubel talks about the need for cultural brokers in Latin America as being of "paramount importance in dual societies, in those nations or regions where two or more culture traditions thrive and where those who provide medical care may be of a different cultural tradition from their patients."[14] Yet, elsewhere in the same article, he points out that Mexican *pasantes*, or those graduate medical students who perform compulsory medical service make "a considerable contribution to the health or rural dwellers in the absence of other facilities," and despite the fact that the overwhelming majority of them do not intend to remain in rural practice and despite the fact that "their socialization and professional training make them even more urbane in outlook and aspirations after graduation than before entering medical school."[15]

What I find objectionable in the writings of so many medical anthropologists and culturally oriented psychiatrists, is not the admirable collection of data, cultural or clinical, which is the only situation wherein we may speak uncompromisingly of the relativity of values, but the *analysis* of the data. Thus, the type of health care that one receives is analyzed *as if* it were a consequence of the culture. All cultures, of course, are good. For therapeutic impotence one substitutes the "natural process of healing" and "knowing the culture" as an expression of clinical therapeutic morality. Williams paper is illustrative here.

If we are relatively sophisticated we tend to think of disease as being multi-causal. And if we are concerned with "mental illness" and are relatively sophisticated, we are definitely multi-causal (psychodynamic) in our thinking. Even the drug companies in their therapy-of-choice advertising recognize multi-causality as they urge one or another of drugs for purposes of "management" or the patient's "productive activity," or "control." After all, what the drug ideally is designed to produce is improvement in thought, affect and behavior in order to help the physician help the patient to get it all together. In short, make the patient more "responsive" to his environment. Indeed, no psychiatric drug can claim a "cure," and only to a certain extent, "symptom control," and "management." The moral-ethical question is, or should be, management of what? Obviously, management of the patient-person in terms of his life. The use of drugs has nothing to do with a "better way of life," a "reactionary," or a "revolutionary" way, etc. It is simply a question of management. Any tranquilizer, etc., can be as much a part of a revolutionary movement as of a conservative movement. It all depends on what the "manager" wants to get across.

I would suggest that the concept of "management" in

relationship to drug efficacy, is very similar to the concept of relativity in cultural description. Just as the tradition of medicine lends itself to reductionism and management, the tradition of cultural relativism lends itself to reductionism and management.

"Management," however, is not a word of choice among psychiatrists and anthropologists who are currently involved with each other in the new interdisciplinary business of health-care. The word-of-choice is "healing." "Management" is manipulative, "healing" somehow is processual. With healing, of course, goes cooperation, between traditional healers and psychiatrists, as urged in the papers by Westermeyer, Williams, Messing, Ruiz, and Araneta. This is the so-called "therapeutic alliance." "Revolution," for healers committed to homeostasis, and anthropologists schooled in cultural relativistic integrity, is obviously not a therapeutic idea. Similarly, "morality" has little or nothing to do with the so-called healing process. Both physicians (and I include psychiatrists here) who are well aware of their limitations, and anthropologists who find a holier-than-thou omnipotence in finding fuctional cultural integrity in all beliefs, including witchcraft, sub-incision, and the value of woodpecker scalps, tend to regard with primitive awe that which their present level of knowledge makes it difficult for them to understand or explain—the healing process, the placebo phenomenon, spontaneous remission.

But what about morality? Can we not say that one thing is better than another? Can we not say that it is better to be healthy and wealthy rather than sick and poor? Can we not say that it is better to be rational than irrational? Can we not say that it is better to believe in the "x" factor of spontaneous remission than that the devil was driven out?

Generally, the anthropologist's highest level of organization, without resorting to a "superorganic," or a Marxist evolutionism, has been the idea of culture, and the moral order and world view to be found within cultures which includes witchcraft, etc. For the eclectic psychiatrist it has been relief of symptoms and restoration of functional integrity.

But if we define colonialism as the imposition of historical and structural variables that occur *outside* the individual and in turn lead to an exploitation of the individual because of the distribution of power, including the power of belief, and the power to maintain belief, then we must forsake the idea of integrative levels, in favor of moral choices. Thus, morality, ethics, becomes the only integrative level which can be thought to be cross-culturally valid.

In psychiatric case conferences, it is not the case presentation, nor the dynamic formulation which is usually most productive of discussion, but the "management" plan. This is so, it seems to me, because the only integrative level that exists for the "liberal" psychiatrist, that is, those of the human potential movement who are most accepting of traditional healers, is that which is good for the individual practitioner, but not necessarily for the patient. Thus, each practitioner imposes his own idiopathic integrative pattern, reflecting his own level of integration and helplessness. So it is that we find psychiatrists like Westermeyer, Ruiz and Araneta, physicians like Williams, and anthropologists like Messing, accepting symptom relief as an end in itself, each one justifying this on the basis of either a biological model or a cultural model.

No one denies the intrinsic value of anthropological knowledge of health and illness behavior. The question is whether or not that cultural knowledge points to the direction of improved human health conditions. I would argue that good health is largely a function of the social and economic conditions that make possible the conditions for good health, i.e., nutrition, housing, water, sewage, etc. I would further argue, with Kroeber, that good health, mental and physical, is a function of the acceptance of the "progress idea."[16] As Kroeber puts it, in presenting his argument for what constitutes a "higher" or more advanced culture, there are three approaches or criteria:

> (1) "In proportion as a culture disengages itself from reliance on (magic and superstition) it may be said to have registered an advance. In proportion as it admits magic in its operations, it remains primitive or retarded. . .[17]

Kroeber's second group of traits characterizing backward as against advanced cultures, has to do

". . . with the obtrusion of physiological or anatomical considerations into social situations, or with the related matter of
the taking of human life."[18]

Here a wide variety of practices are included, ranging from
puberty crisis rites to animal sacrifice.

The third criteria Kroeber posits as an objective approach
to the idea of progress in culture

". . ,can be justified by objective evidence. This is in technology,
mechanics, and science, whose accomplishments have definitely more cumulative quality than other civilizational
activities."[19]

Medicine, as a scientific discipline, certainly demonstrates progress over the last 100 years in these very areas.
Psychiatry, particularly so-called cross-cultural psychiatry
and its hand-maiden, medical anthropology, demonstrates
the opposite with its insistence on "using" the traditional
healer. By insisting on the integrity, and the power of the
culture concept, psychiatry, as a branch of medicine, neatly
avoids[20] the issue of health care in a socio-economic setting.

But, "knowing the culture" rarely becomes a vehicle
for a social change strategy for the powerless in the culture.
Obviously, to manipulate the culture in such a way as to give
power to the powerless, in terms of access to services and resources, is political, and political is taboo for most anthropologists because it involves changing power relationships.
As for the medical anthropologist, he has always been part
of the professional team, and as such his contribution is to
things as they are, rather than to change, to working with the
culture as if it were a problem in methodology-technology,
rather than a problem of values and politics. Looked at in
this way, the so-called "clinical judgement" whether to
admit or not to admit, to prescribe or not prescribe, to call
in a traditional healer, or a social worker; to refer or not to
refer; to intervene or not to intervene, etc., all break down
into a series of questions and issues which can be analyzed on
the basis of values and goals.

But, if one is a physician, and clinical decisions are to be based on something other than clinical aspects of a problem, then what is one to do? Use the "cultural" knowledge of the traditional healer, suggest Drs. Araneta, Ruiz and Westermeyer. But, is cultural judgement the same as clinical judgement? I would submit it is not, and to confuse cultural behavior with the clinical alteration of behavior is as an error as to confuse the functional with the organic. To talk about the traditional healer, or the paraprofessional, or the non-professional, as if he were an aspect of "health manpower" is to further confuse the realities of the value choices and problems. Discourse and data may be value free, but clinical judgement and therapy, that is, doing something to someone, is not. This problem is particularly acute in the so-called mental, or functional illness cases where the sick role model as it exists in organic illness becomes antitherapeutic in mental illness. The "sick role" in Western organic medicine absolves the individual from his usual cultural behavior obligations, and once "sick" he is no longer a person, but a disease in a chart. In trying to transfer this model to the mental patient, the therapist has discovered that he can only do so at the peril of the patient's health. The value of the traditional healer approach, well brought out by Mume, Mburu and Lambo, is that the person is not seen as a sick role patient, but is still valued as a person within the norms of the culture. He is as he was before, except in certain behavioral areas where cultural events such as broken taboos, witchcraft, spirit possession, have been at work against him. Behavioral homeostasis is restored through cultural event manipulation, usually in the community. The Western mental patient, however, under the organic sick role model, is no longer a person, but a patient, not responsible for himself, and most likely to be restored to his "normal" (not cultural) self through the use of extrinsic, organic, usually drug treatment of disease. If the sulfas and penicillin and other antibiotics could do wonders for the organically sick, then certainly the antipsychotic drugs would do the trick for the "other" diseases. Indeed, this is now the position of the United States National Institute of Mental Health which has recently reported that one of every ten Americans suffers from mental illness and that drugs are the

16

best means of combatting it. This obviously puts the "culturally" oriented practitioner into a bind. Like Doctor Araneta, he knows the value of psychotropic drugs and electroconvulsive therapy, but yet his cultural "clinical" experience has also taught him something about the density of the cultural experience and the need to work with cultural events. It is this "density" or cultural complexity, which makes the problem of diagnosis so difficult, and without appropriate diagnosis, how is one to prescribe the appropriate drug? Well, given that kind of doubt, one uses the traditional healer in conjunction *with* the drug. But what is it then that works? Cultural manipulation/reinforcement, or the drug? That kind of clinical data is apparently not available.

Where traditional healers do possess an extensive herbal pharmacopeia, it may also explain their general indifference to the question of dose levels which is constantly put to them by sympathetic and cultural Westerners. Chief Lambo is very sensitive to, and critical of, the statements that the traditional healers do not possess standard dosages. He need not be, since dosage in the psychotropic drugs is so variable and individual "that the only rational method for judging dosage in any individual patient is to titrate the desired therapeutic effect against the unwanted effects."[21] This may explain in part the great reluctance I have encountered on the part of major drug companies to run the kind of clinical studies, using traditional drugs and treatment, that they run in America and then use to promote their chemical analogs. How embarrasing it would be to find out that the herb of choice of the traditional healer is indeed effective. Of course, there would be no easy way to eliminate the cultural context, and, as representatives of drug companies have told me, "herbs are not patentable." Nevertheless, psychiatrists who consider themselves cross-cultural researchers, sensitive and sympathetic to the cultural milieu, persist in the perpetuation of the notion of mental illness." For example, Ari Kiev writes:

> To the extent that indigenous forms of treatment are effective, the extent of psychiatric illness in any given community will tend to be underestimated. Some individuals who receive help

17

within a religious context will not be identified as cases, even in the most rigorous of community surveys. Others, satisfied with the results of the indigenous healer, have little urge to consult modern medical facilities. [22]

As clinicians, whether Western, or traditional, healers must deal with the individual. The pharmacological anarchy cited above is a reflection of Western medical capitalism-colonialism that refuses to go beyond the stressed individual for the cause and cure of diseases. The traditional cultural event of the traditional healer is precisely its colonial counterpart in its refusal to countenance the kind of progress which would threaten traditional prerogatives, as Mburu points out. It is no accident that the severest critic of the traditional healers comes from an African, Mburu, himself the son of a traditional healer, who is trained in public health. This is the one medical discipline which understands the relation of the individual to the society. In that sense, it can be called anti-colonial, even Marxist. It is also no accident that public health enjoys the lowest esteem among the physician class in America. It also tends to receive minimal support in newly developing countries. They may help to partially explain Mburu's ambivalence resulting in a quasi-endorsement of the "duality" of the two systems. We "live and let live" under conditions of affluent pluralism and overwhelming under-development.

Dawkins, in his typology of the "indigenous healers" in the South Bronx, makes it very clear that the creation of most of these healers is due to the type of colonialism people in the South Bronx live under. He does not have the great rationalizing, justifying argument of "traditional culture" to give credence to these types, and so he is full of anger.

Messing's paper on traditional healing in Ethiopia is the traditional anthropologist's paper and stands out in marked contrast to the Dawkins' contribution by its "outsider" stance and uncommitted manner. In stressing as he does, the "syndrome of difficulties" in the provision of health care in Ethiopia, Messing assumes that I would call the "I'm just an anthropologist (housewife)" role. The paper by Ruiz and Langrod needs to be read in conjunction with that of the Dawkins' to most clearly see the issues delineated of "getting along" versus Revolution.

The danger, however, is that so-called "psychiatric disorders" will come to be seen as public health disorders. Indeed, Kiev urges that it be looked at that way:

> Much as penicillin and anti-malarial drugs have facilitated nationwide campaigns to eradicate yaws and malaria, the psychopharmaceuticals can be used in a public health approach to psychiatric disorders. . .To the extent. . .that psychiatry is concerned with fundamental human issues that are central to the political and economic stability of developing societies, it is imperative that such programs be established as a first and major priority.[23]

One of the results of that approach is exemplified in the chapter by Ruiz and Landgrod in this book. Dawkins presents the opposing view.

All underdeveloped countries that I know of, while citing the need for more physicians, still cite the fact that what physicians they have are concentrated in the urban areas. There we see at once the survivals of colonialism and contradictions and antagonisms in a social system. Many underdeveloped, independent countries export physicians. This "brain drain" is due to the fact that the countries in question are still colonial in system. The biggest exporters I have personal knowledge of are India and the Phillipines. Another exporter is Guyana. In all these countries, folk medicine and traditional healing are very powerful. Pre-revolutionary Cuba was also an exporter of physicians. It is thus somewhat ironic that Dr. Ruiz, a Cuban, should advocate a closer link between folk healers and professional mental health workers for Hispanic patients. It is particularly ironic because Dr. Ruiz himself coined the term "environmental oppression" to explain many of the mental health problems encountered in the South Bronx. Nevertheless, he still advocates attention to the hispanic's cultural background, including belief in the supernatural, voodoo and spiritualism, instead of environmental revolution.

The major distinction between traditional and psychiatric healing and science as a methodology, is that traditional healing, etc., is basically a mediation or "brokerage" process between the individual and the dominant values, institutions, powers, agencies, etc., that exist and with which he has to cope. There is nothing transcendent about it, as there is about science as a method. Its major focus is adaptation and maladaptation. It is only natural then, as Ruiz points out, that folk healers can do better than psychiatrists in "therapeutic" approaches. Folk healers are closer to the mediating street savvy needed to exist. In a ghetto society the folk healers do indeed make possible appropriate "acting out" not favored by the larger society. It is no coincidence that the healing function in colonial societies remains closely linked to the priestly offices, while science is divorced from religion by and large. What is basic to all the colonial, i.e., traditional modes of therapy, and indeed to colonialism itself, is the fact of dependency upon authority.

What Ruiz, Mume, Lambo, Messing all have in common is apparently a belief in the magical and irrational self "cured" by making the individual, through the mediation of the healer, once again into a member of the culture, that is the colonial culture.

The fact that this is achieved through psychiatric processes such as acting out, catharsis, abreaction, rituals, etc., does not, however, lend it to any more rationalism for all that. It is still a performance of dependency. The fact that anthropologists and psychiatrists seek to rationalize dependency through process, does not make it any more acceptable, but even more disgusting (sic) because these are people who presumably know better. But, as Messing wrote to me, when I asked him to revise his paper:

> . . .I don't see what purpose can be served by denouncing 'failure' in stronger terms.

I would maintain that what would once have been accepted during another cultural time, when persons of power believed that there was indeed a superordinate world of mystical powers and values and magico-religious forces, a world that went beyond colonialism, that belief no longer exists in the age of a handshake in space between Apollo and

Soyuz, and to insist it does is to do a disservice to persons in need, not of soul salvation, but higher levels of living.

Thus, far from being either therapists or culture describers, the alliance between psychiatrists and anthropologists has become the alliance of "mediatorial elites."[24] Without ever facing up to the questions of values and morality, they pretend to mediate or "broker" between suffering persons and a mystical world now defined as the "Healing Process," or, in the case of anthropologists, the reality of cultural differences.

As part of the new mediatorial elites, anthropologists and psychiatrists join hands, no longer perhaps in the cure of souls through the instrumentalities of divination, exorcism, absolution, ritual, revealing, etc., but in the new Gnostic movements of the Human Potential Movements, and Roche Laboratories "The Natural Processes of Healing" with an assist from Valium.

It is important to emphasize that when we speak of the "therapeutic alliance" we are speaking primarily about *psychiatrists* and traditional healers, not the primary physicians. This is largely because the anxieties and psychosomatic illnesses in particular are successfully treated by traditional healers, or so-called "folk medicine."[25]

It is largely for this same reason that psychiatry has flourished in the West. The primary physician is dealing with organic problems. I want to urge that it *is* necessary to again separate mind and body when thinking of the delivery of health care services. The psychosomatic continuum stressed by modern physicians is a luxury which underdeveloped societies cannot afford, either in terms of physicians who are psychiatrists, or in the employ of witchdoctors or other traditional healers who serve to maintain the same belief system which made colonialism possible in the first instance.

Anthropologists and psychiatrists again and again make the point that the illnesses of other cultures can only be understood within the context of its own social system and milieu, and that it is useless to try to apply Western psychiatric diagnostic categories.

That is precisely the point. It is the social system that perpetuates certain psychosomatic diseases, and when that

21

system is colonial in practice, in terms of exploitation, etc., it is necessary to recognize it as such and try to do something about the system and not the disease.

Without some integrating moral imperatives beyond the culture of the anthropologists, or the symptom relief of the psychiatrists, we can get into some truly ridiculous, self-justifying situations. For example, Kennedy (Kennedy, J.C., "Psychosocial Dynamics of Witchcraft Systems," *International Journal of Social Psychiatry*, 90, 1970) and Dobkin de Rios in an unpublished paper ("Witchcraft and Psychosomatic Illness"), discuss witchcraft in terms of disease patterning and cure, as highly adaptive from an ecological point of view, because "a population which has grown beyond the resources of its environment may fission and set up a new village due to witchcraft fear." (Dobkin de Rios)

The question must be asked—which is to be preferred, village fissioning due to witchcraft fears, or population control on a rational basis?

A major part of the problem for Nigeria and other independent African countries *is that they already have their independence* and therefore do not have any ideological or strategical grounds for professionalizing reforms within the traditional system. Whereas revolutionary values were once progress and reform and cultural identity, independence values, at least as put forth by Chief Lambo, seem to be a return to the traditional values of acceptance of traditional systems without question. Face-to-face with the enemy, the white colonial master, one could argue the necessity for the return to African traditional healing culture, especially since the colonial medicine was primarily for the colonial expatriates. But, now face-to-face with his own free Black Brother and Sister, it would appear that the Black Traditional Healer has the same compulsion to exploit, as even his colonial master did. The tradition which his revolution called upon him to legitimate, to affirm, no longer is as urgent in independence, as the need to provide legitimate service. It is no longer valid to argue in free times, as in colonial times, that Western doctors are few in number, and therefore it was the traditional healers in the rural areas who were serving the needs of the people. Now it is time to provide the best possible service to all the peoples by professionalizing the services of the traditional healers, if they were willing. Where the colonial master could once contemptuously dismiss the traditional healer by asserting that they best suited the un-developed racial evolutionary character of the rural masses, this argument cannot, and should not be made by the free African or American. Medicine, qua organic medicine, is as good for you as it is for me. However, medicine, qua functional symbolism, is another matter, and there I am prepared to acknowledge the efficacy of one symbolic system over another.

Indeed, this is about as far as I am prepared to go in defense of cultural relativism. Whatever you think and believe is fine and I will not argue with you. However, what you *do* about what you think and believe is another matter. If your belief system leads you to a system of ante-natal and birth delivery care that results in a high rate of infant mortality, I am opposed to it; if your belief system leads you to accept fees for forecasting and astrological diagnosis that you your-self do not believe in, I am opposed to it; if your belief system leads you to prescribe herbal remedies while keeping the information about your materia medica secret, I am opposed to it; if your belief system leads you to condemn a neighbor for practicing witchcraft on a person suffering from "bad luck," I am opposed to it; if your belief system leads you to prescribe drugs needlessly for a so-called "anxiety state" because you will be reimbursed by third-party payment, I am opposed to it.

Physicians have long known that ethical judgements are part of clinical judgements. Anthropologists are not so sure that data collection and analysis may also represent a problem in ethical judgement. The problem seems to lie in the fact that although organic illnesses which can be treated and cured by organic (physical) means are readily thera-peutically transferable and acceptable cross-culturally, the so-called functional, or mental disorders are more difficult to cope with cross-culturally and within the prevailing thera-peutic armamentarium. Whether or not someone is "mentally ill" seems to involve a philosophical and cultural question as to the "nature" of people. For the physician turned psychiatrist, it means he is no longer a physician treating organic illnesses, but basically a blunderer, not sure of what he is doing or why, but governed by the medical model.

For the anthropologist turned mental health clinician-helper-therapist-broker, it means that he has crossed the threshhold of dependent participant-observer, helpless and humble before the complexity of total immersion in another culture; to arrogant [26] helper—his traditional helplessness and dependency on the people he is living with turned around so that he is again powerful—therapeutic, and to that extent, colonialist. The field dependency situation is completely turned about in the medical anthropologist setting, especially in psychiatric hospitals and community mental health centers in his own culture. The shift from field problems of transference-counter-transference to structured relations of dependency, the patient upon the anthropologist-therapist, is fairly complete, and the conviction by the anthropologist of his absolute therapeutic goodness grows and grows. His fight now is to share power with the psychiatrist, in order to provide "culturally appropriate" therapy.

NOTES

[1]On this point, see Lewis, D., "Anthropology and Colonialism", *Current Anthropology*, V. 14, No. 5, Dec. 1973, pp. 581-602.

[2]Morgan, D.H., "Psychotherapy of Jealousy," *Psychother. Psychosom.*, 25:43-47, 1975, as reported in *Psychiatry Digest*, July, 1975, p. 11.

[3]Perhaps the best, or worst, example of the "clinical" anthropologist is to be found in the writings of medical anthropologist Joan Halifax-Grof. In a paper presented to the American Anthropological Association, New Orleans, 1973, she and her psychiatrist husband, Stanislav Grof, discuss using LSD with terminal cancer patients. Dr. Joan Halifax-Grof writes about how she "works with a dying individual. . .in much the same way as one would relate to an informant in the field." She apparently sees no conflict in her role as anthropologist and therapist, and in her discussions with the dying patients "to the idea of the continuity of consciousness after physical demise, the soul's survival of death, or the concept of reincarnation." Xerox paper: "LSD-Assisted Psychotherapy with Terminal Cancer Patients: Anthropological Perspectives."

[4]Willner, D., "Anthropology: Vocation or Commodity?" In *Current Anthropology*, V. 14, No. 5, Dec. 1973, pp. 547-555.

[5]Simpson, G., *The Meaning of Evolution*, Yale University Press, New Haven, 1949.

[6]Gardner, E.A., "Serving an Urban Ghetto Through a Community Mental Health Center," *Mental Health Program Reports*, No. 4, January 1970, pp. 69-106.

[7]*Ibid.*, p. 87.

[8]*Ibid.*, p. 83.

[9]*Ibid.*, p. 83

[10]Redlich, F.C., "The Concept of Normality," *American Journal of Psychotherapy*, No. 6, 1952, pp. 551-568.

[11]Gardner, *op. cit.*, p. 84.

[12]Arnhoff, F.N., "Social Consequences of Policy Toward Mental Illness," *Science*, 27 June 1975.

[13]Cited in *Hospital Tribune*, April 21, 1975, p. 4.

[14]Rubel, A. J., "Social Science and Health Research in Latin America," *The Milbank Memorial Fund Quarterly*, No. 2, April 1968, Part 2, pp. 21-33, p. 27.

[15]*Ibid.*, p. 25.

[16]Kroeber, A., *Anthropology*. Harcourt, Brace and Co., N.Y., 1948, esp. pp. 296-304.

[17]*Ibid.*, p. 298.

[18]*Ibid.*, p. 300.

[19]*Ibid.*, p. 303.

[20]A good example of this type of "avoidance" behavior is to be found in Kiev, A., *Transcultural Psychiatry*, The Free Press, N.Y., 1972.

[21]Blackwell, B., "Rational Drug Use in Psychiatry." In *Rational Psychopharmacoltherapy and the Right to Treatment*, Ayd, F.J., Jr., (ed.) Ayd Medical Communications, Lts., Baltimore, Md. 1974, pp. 187-199, p. 191.

[22]Kiev, A., *Transcultural Psychiatry*. The Free Press, New York. 1972, p. 139.

[23]Kiev, *op. cit.*, p. 166.

[24]See Nelson, B., "Mental Healers and Their Philosophies," *Psychoanalytic Review*, 52, No. 2, Summer 1965, pp. 131-136.

[25]Kiev, A., *Magic, Faith and Healing*, N.Y., Free Press, 1964.

[26]For a good example of this kind of arrogance and presumption of therapeutic knowledge, see *Psychiatric Annals*, Special Issue on "Psychiatry and the Social Sciences," V. 5, No. 8, August 1975. The issue is devoted to the work of the Department of Psychiatry, University of Miami School of Medicine, and the Community Mental Health Service of the Mental Health Services Division of Jackson Memorial Hospital. It is largely devoted to a discussion of providing "culturally appropriate" mental health care.

THE RELIGIOUS COMPONENT IN SOUTHERN FOLK MEDICINE

Loudell F. Snow, Ph.D.

I've seen paralyzed people *walk,* I've seen the blind to *see,* I've seen *diseased cleansed.* I have been healed myself. I don't know if I had polio or what it was. It was very painful; my neck, I couldn't move it. And I was weak, I weakened down in nothin' flat. Like in two days I was weakened down I couldn't eat, I couldn't sleep. All I did was moan and cry and I couldn't move. *And,* I don't know if you've ever heard of anointed handkerchiefs? The church anointed a handkerchief and prayed all night and I got over it. The oil, it's olive oil, actually, prayer oil. They just soak the handkerchief in it and pray over it. Then they bring it and place it on the afflicted. You don't have to be in the same *room,* they just went back to the church and prayed. Prayer meeting.

And through the night, I just, I don't know, I just *felt* it! When they placed it on me I couldn't hardly talk. When they placed it on me they asked me if I believed that through Jesus Christ my Saviour I could be *healed* and bein' a child I believed because they told me I could if I believed. And of course when it was all over with the next morning I was well.

And I was taken to the hospital when it first happened and they wasn't sure what it was. And at that time polio was a wild thing. And that hospital there, bein' country as it was, they wasn't sure. They took some tests but they wasn't real positive. At that time polio was *new* (1954), it wasn't a old disease. They wasn't sure enough to put me *in* the hospital, they didn't know what to do with me if they *did.* So they sent me back home and the church *healed* me. I have seen many, many afflictions prayed for, healed. And I really believe if you *believe,* it'll *happen!* It's through the power of believing and through asking Greater Sources, Greater Powers, and believing in Greater Powers. And I was healed.[1]

The speaker of the above words is a young housewife and mother of three, born and raised in the coal mining region of West Virginia. She comes from a health culture where being a seventh son lends more credence to the status "doctor" than would a diploma from Harvard Medical School. Her statements are of the type likely to make the health professional wince and the faithful smile—no practitioner will ever convince her that, polio or not, she was not healed by the prayer handkerchief. Frank has pointed out that the apparent success of non-medical healing techniques "...seems to lie in their ability to arouse the patient's hope, bolster his self-esteem, stir him emotionally, and strengthen his ties with a supportive group, through several features that most methods share. All involve a healer on whom the patient depends for help and who holds out hope of relief. The patient's expectations are aroused by the healer's personal attributes, by his culturally determined healing role, or, typically, by both."[2] At least one writer has suggested, in fact, that the witchdoctor and the psychiatrist are but cultural variations of the same person and that treatment outcomes are about the same for *good* therapists worldwide.[3] Most physicians, however, would share the puzzlement expressed by the, "But she seems to be an *intelligent* woman," which a practitioner kept repeating as he told of a black woman who refused the surgical removal of uterine fibroids.[4] The patient in question insisted just as firmly that God would heal her if it were His will. It was her belief in "faith healing" which caused the surgeon to question her IQ.

To many the term faith healing is likely to call up a mental picture of the wild-eyed evangelist, the revival attended by the ignorant and superstitious, the tortured last resort of the incurably ill, the throwing away of crutches by the credulous. The medical establishment has viewed such cures in a variety of ways ranging from open derision to thoughtful attempts to explain how putative cures actually work. The former view, however, is probably the more prevalent. Hippocrates himself is credited with wishing to find a natural explanation for the "sacred disease" (epilepsy) and for railing against "...the sort of people we now call witch-doctors, faith-healers, quacks and charlatans."[5] In contrast, a British psychiatrist searched unsuccessfully for twenty years for an "...irrefutable cure...not in the vague sense of a patient's 'feeling better' or even in that a progressive disease had been limited, but in the sense that, as a result of the healer's work alone, a demonstrable pathological state had been entirely eliminated."[6] An American physician has even more recently made a similar search for a real miracle cure with similar results, i.e., no cures in which some other explanation could not be brought to bear (ranging from out-and-out fakery to psychogenic factors.)[7] Such findings do not convince the faithful, of course. To the true believer an N of 1 is sufficient as far as miracles are concerned and you certainly do not subject the Almighty to double blind studies. This emphasis on the dramatic tends to obscure the more mundane part that religion plays in traditional folk medical belief, however. It is as if one attempted to describe modern scientific medicine by speaking only of emergency surgical interventions and the intensive care unit. In this sense, that is, the miracle cure is the heart transplantation of folk medicine. This is unfortunate in that most attention is paid to the last ditch effort to obtain a cure while ignoring the *weltanschauung* that makes such action natural and understandable. If the physician comprehends that for many people *all healing* is faith healing the decision not to have surgery may at least be rational if no less regrettable. Quite literally, in fact, the very decision to take an aspirin for a headache may be seen as divinely inspired. Then,

> If you should go to the doctor, I think God has directed you or your *mind*, you know, to go to the doctor. Cause I feel that God has given these doctors knowledge to help people and to cure them. Sometimes I feel your healing has come from both: that God has given them the *knowledge*, and that He give you the *faith*. In this doctor and in Him.[8]

The remainder of this paper will focus on the underlying religious motif which directs so much of the life of the poor rural Southerner, white or black, whether still living "down home" or having migrated to northern or western urban centers. Information presented comes from both published sources and my own ethnographic research (I should like to emphasize that my research has *not* been directed to religion *per se;* rather, the focus has been on folk medical belief and the religious element was inescapable.)[9]

Most informants come from areas which demonstrate what folklorist Richard Dorson would call the "...classical elements of the folk community...isolation, illiteracy, mar-

ginal living, close contact with nature,"[10] i.e., eastern
Kentucky, the Southern Appalachians and the Ozarks. To
such people folk cures mean ". . .faith in tradition, faith in
the fact that 'my grandmother told me,' faith that it worked
for a neighbor and can or may work for me."[11] The
conceptual distance between folk and scientific medicine can
only be widened when there is cultural approval for accepting
symptoms stoically, when a feeling of "dullishness" is usual,
when "feeling sick" is expected.[12,13] The problem is
exacerbated by the view that it is almost shameful to go to
the doctor, that symptoms ought to be "punished out," when
there is disdain for those who "give in" and seek professional
care, when people are apologetic about such visits, saying,
"I'm funny about that," or, "We're bad to run to the
doctor."[14,15] Unfortunately, too often the decision to seek
medical help ends in a mutually unsatisfactory encounter
which reinforces the common view that doctors are only
interested in treating the "higher ups":

> I tried a lot of different methods of my own with the
> baby because he had the colic. He was a newborn baby
> and I finally just wore out; he cried from four in the
> evenin' 'til four in the morning.' You know how colicky
> babies are; you cain't lay 'em down. The heat of the
> mother kind of soothes their cramps; you just hold 'em
> and rock and rock. I was exhausted, you know, after just
> havin' a baby you are wore out anyhow and you don't
> have that kind of strength. So I took him in with the colic,
> and I told the doctor, "This young'un is just woolin' me to
> death!" He laughed and says, "What do you mean by that?"
> And *he* thought it was *funny!* He didn't know what I
> meant by "woolin'" and *I* didn't know that he didn't
> know! He said, "I don't understand that word "woolin',""
> and I said, "Well, that means aggravatin', buggin' me,
> botherin' me." And *he* said, "Well, this hillbilly talk I just
> don't understand."[1]

The preceding attitudes provide a fertile ground for the
retention of traditional beliefs and for a world view which
emphasizes the importance of external supernatural sources
of help. This theme of personal helplessness is exemplified in
such spirituals as the popular Without the Lord I Could Do
Nothing: 'Without the Lord I could do nothing. . .I couldn't
walk. . .I couldn't talk. . .I couldn't see. . .I couldn't be."[17]

Many of the rural and urban poor belong to churches of a fundamentalist and pentecostal nature in which the religious experience is intense and passionate.[18-21] They emphasize a personalized relationship with God and a literal interpretation of the Bible. A firmly stated, "It's in the Bible," is considered the last word on any topic, including medical care. Healing, in fact, is a regularly scheduled part of services in such churches and a particular scriptural passage is frequently cited as the basis for such rituals (James 5:14-17):

> If one of you is ill, he should send for the elders of the church, and they must anoint him with oil in the name of the Lord and pray over him. The prayer of faith will save the sick man and the Lord will raise him up again; and if he has committed any sins, he will be forgiven. So confess your sins to one another, and pray for one another, and this will cure you; the heartfelt prayer of a good man works very powerfully.

Good health is seen as being a gift from God, a gift enjoyed by few. Poor health is also explained from a spiritual standpoint—certainly God "allows" illness and other misfortune. Frequently such events are seen as being direct punishment for sin:

> Seem like a lot of times things come through Him like that; lot of times people will be well. And then on down the line somethin' will happen to him, sometimes be crippled. And then be out workin' around machinery sometimes, somethin' will explode. Cause him to lose his sight, accidental things. So many different things, for sinnin' all the time. We here in the world sin. Things gonna come upon us, unless we serve Him more. I think if we go away from Him, He might suffer some of these things to happen.[8]

There is a particular emphasis on the death, deformity or retardation of children as being the result of sinful parents:

> I feel that a lot of things that you do, when you're disobedient to God's will, that a curse or something is put on you. . .sometimes I think it could be in the form of an illness. To really say, sometime I think retarded children is a curse, and that's something you've got to go through for the rest of their life or your life. They say somewhere in the Bible about you can be whipped by many stripes. I think that person has been whipped till he has come to his knowledge of his sins and knowing that he was sinful. Then it make him a better person or made him closer to God.[8]

30

Sometimes, of course, constant misfortune is the lot of a *good* person, the rationale here being that God is testing the individual's faith.

When health problems of either a minor or serious nature do occur the illness referral system is affected similarly by religious belief. For any health problem the best remedies are those seen as being "natural" ones, i.e., plants and herbs. Several informants pointed out that herbs are mentioned in the very first book of the Bible, signaling the Almighty's intention that they should be used for medicine.[22] Furthermore, " 'God Almighty never put us here without a remedy for every ailment,' said old Jimmy Van Zandt of Kirbyville, Missouri. 'Out in the woods there's plants that will cure all kinds of sickness, and all we got to do is hunt for 'em!'."[23] Herbal remedies are still very important to many although their use may be deliberately hidden from health professionals who might laugh at such "old timey" remedies.[24-25] It is expected, in fact, that everyone know something of the various medicinal plants of an area and their proper uses. Some people may gain the reputation of knowing more than most, however, and become an "herb doctor," or "yarb doctor." One informant's father had been called "the Daddy of the Herbs." Not only was his special talent seen as a gift from God but his cures were often the result of divine revelation:

> When we was small, why, he'd get a hard case of some kind. And most places where we lived was a fireplace, you know, and a chimley. And he'd take a chair, they had chairs then with shuck bottoms—do you know about them? They used to use the thick comforters, they called 'em. He'd fold one of them and spread it down. . . .across in front of the fireplace on the floor. And he'd take one of them shuck-bottom chairs and he'd turn it down with the back of it down, and he'd let the quilt come up onta that. And he'd lay down on it flat on his back, and he'd fold his arms and shet his eyes. And we knowed to be quiet. And sometime we'd be playin', you know, runnin' and runnin' and hoppin' and playin', and we'd leap over his feet.
> He'd have his eyes shut, but he wouldn't be asleep. Ever once in awhile he'd say, "Ooooooh, Lordy!" And he'd go on awhile, "Thank you, Lord!" Just like that. And he'd get up. He'd say, "Sister, you come along and go with me. The Lord showed me some more roots to dig.[8]

His talents allowed him to make a full time living and earned him the appellation "doctor," as well.

There are a number of different kinds of folk healers of which the herb doctor is but one example. There are tremendous variations in kinds of healer, how they are believed to have received the power to heal, what sorts of things they can cure and the techniques utilized. They share one thing in common, however, and that is that their ability is a gift from God. There are three general ways to classify folk healers in the rural Southern tradition, 1) they learned their craft, 2) they received ability during an altered state of consciousness, or, 3) they were born with the power to heal. Healers also tend to be ranked according to the amount of power they possess and this is loosely correlated with how it was allocated—as in most traditional societies ascribed statuses outrank achieved ones (the reverse, of course, from modern practitioners). All, however, can be termed shamanistic curers in the broad sense of ". . .any kind of curer or medical *cum* religious practitioner whose powers come from supernaturals."[26]

Power Doctors: Bloodstopping and Firedrawing

Other than herb doctors, the commonest of the achieved healing statuses is the ability to stop bleeding and to remove the pain from burns. Such ability may be referred to as "powwowing," "conjuring," or simply as "having the Power." Both techniques employ the recitation of a verbal charm with religious overtones. The commonest verse to stop blood by is from the Bible, in fact (Ezekiel 16:6):

> And when I passed by thee, and saw thee polluted in thine own blood, I said unto thee *when thou wast* in thy blood, Live; yea, I said unto thee *when thou wast* in thy blood, Live.

And in most folklore in the European tradition the numbers three or its multiple nine are likely to be used. The verse, that is, is likely to be recited three times. The victim's name may also be incorporated in order to personalize the ritual. Bloodstopping by such techniques has been reported since the 13th century.[27] It may be used for bleeding of any sort from that of minor cuts to heavy post-partum bleeding. For the latter Murphree reports one of the rare deviations from the biblical verse, given to her in the following handwritten version: "Stand blood, don't spread, over our land, God the Father, God the Sun (sic), and the Holy Ghost ask it in the name of our Lord Savior, Jesus Christ. Amen."[16] Generally the bloodstopping verses can be taught only to someone of the opposite sex who is not a member of your family. [23,11, 23,28,29,30-34,10] The number three is occasionally incorporated into the number of persons that can be taught or the number of times the charm can be used without losing the power to be effective. One of my informants tried it at the onset of her first menses, not having been forwarned of the event. It did not work but she has since used it with success:

> I'm a very religious-minded person; I know all the stuff for healing, I've been taught. The bloodstopping, I know that. I know the one for drawing the fire. It's about the same one. I cain't tell a woman, I can tell a man and the man can tell a woman. . .I still use it. But you have to use the full name of the person in the verse. You use the full name of the person and then you use the verse. All you do is just *believe yourself!*[1]

Another of my informants once told me how she had used the verse to stop bleeding of a deep cut on a neighborhood boy while at the same time applying ice to the wound. When I asked how she didn't know the ice had not stopped the bleeding she reprimanded me obliquely—and gently—with, "God sewed it with *His* needle, darlin'."[35]

The charm for firedrawing also combines elements of the number three and of sharing it only with a non-family member of the opposite sex.[23,25,28] In this version one blows on the burn while mentally reciting, "Two little angels come from the West—One named Fire and one named Frost, Go away Fire! Come, Frost!."[29] Other versions are, "Out fire, In frost, In the name of Father, Son, and Holy Ghost," or, "Under clod, Under clay, God Almighty take the fire away."[11] The bloodstopping and firedrawing charms are by far the most common, though Randolph cites one intended to drive out intestinal worms.[23]

Another rare but fascinating learned role is the "power to scatter risin's," (i.e., smooth away boils or abscesses by rubbing with the hand) reported by Murphree.[16] The power can be gained by a man who smothers a live mole to death with his bare hands. Perhaps imitative magic is present in the resemblance of molehills to "risings;" it could then be postulated that smothering the life from the mole would remove the abscess. In any case, all that is required of any of the possessors of the above powers (presuming that the rules concerning gender and relationship have been followed) is the ability to learn, to be a "good-hearted" person willing to help others, and, most importantly, to have faith.

Altered States of Consciousness

The power to cure being gained by experiencing an altered state of consciousness is a mixture of achieved and ascribed statuses and is found worldwide. They are achieved in that the individual may actively seek such experiences as when a member of a pentecostal congregation strives to "be filled with the Holy Spirit" for the first time. Henceforth such "falling out" or "getting happy" is a normal part of church services, although it may not always occur. [17-36] Such states are not approved outside of the religious context, however, and may be considered abnormal if they occur elsewhere.[37] In general, altered states of consciousness "...may be produced in any setting by any agents or maneuvers which interfere with the normal outflow of motor impulses, the normal 'emotional tone,' or the normal flow and organization of recognitive processes. There seems to be an optimal range of exteroceptive stimulation necessary for the maintenance of normal, waking consciousness, and levels of stimulation either above or below this range appear conducive to the production of ASC's."[38] Having attended many pentecostal church services I would say that in this case it is stimuli *above* the normal range which is responsible for this phenomenon—with the singing, rhythmic handclapping, call-and-response activity between preacher and congregation and the shouts of the faithful, the excitement—and the din—is incredible. Simpson has studied ecstatic behavior in a St. Louis church and found that "falling out" was most likely to occur during singing by the choir or during preaching, especially if the sermon topic was interpersonal relationships.[17]

Not all individuals who achieve the ability to experience such trance states become healers, of course. Occasionally, however, the Lord selects an individual on whom to confer special powers of healing. Such recruitment is quite similar to that of the shaman as described in the anthropological literature in that 1) the individual is personally selected by the supernatural (in this case, God), 2) the "call" usually occurs during a trance or vision, 3) the healer cooperates with the supernatural during the healing ritual, i.e., is the vessel through which power flows and, 4) is often only a part time specialist. Frequently "the call" comes to fundamentalist Christians during the special excitement of a religious revival, as in the following example:

> I was called by God! Darlin', He called me one mornin' and give me my position. To visit the sick and to preach and to help save the laws. And I heard this and I didn't believe it! I went on back to sleep, and then He woke me up again. And this mellow-toned voice, you know, waked me again. And I wasn't frightened, it wasn't a frightenin' voice, it was a *glorious* voice! I don't know whether you ever felt the Lord or not. When I felt the Lord, it just woke me out of sleep, just seem like it touched me all over. And called me by my name: "Erma! Go ye therefore!" I said, "Yes, Lord." . . .It was one mornin' afore day. God called me to a ministry. And to visit the sick and pray for the sick, and pray for the hands that handles them and so forth. . . .That night when He called me to a ministry here, it meant somethin' in life to me. I mean it *meant* that I couldn't stop, wherever I go. If I went to Kansas, I went in the hospitals there, too. He gave me somethin' in my hands that I could touch the peoples that they may be healed.[35]

It is quite common for such individuals also to become licensed ministers as well, which not only confers high status in the group but offers some protection against charges of practicing medicine without a license. These are the people who best fit the stereotype conjured up by the term "faith healer"—they are thought by the faithful to be able to cure illnesses beyond the power of the physician:

> See, now, if you have cancer, the doctors can't cure cancer! But if they go prayin' for you, and you have lots of faith, the Lord will cure that cancer! The Lord heals a whole lot of people of things the doctors done give up! While the doctor may give you up, the Lord can come in and deliver you! Put you on your feet! Then whenever the doctor come back and examine you for that particular thing and he don't see it, why, he'll say, "Well, I know it was there, but I don't know what became of you now!" They'll be amazed theirself; they want to know what happened."[35]

It may be said that the Lord does such things to cause others to have more faith.[39]

Born with the Power

Certain high statuses, including the power to heal, are ascribed at birth or even before. This infers, of course, that the infant must be somehow identifiable in the prenatal period or at birth as usual. One of the most common of such instances is the Man Who Has Never Seen His Father (i.e., a male child born after the death of his father.) Such a person is usually reported as being able to cure only one illness, most commonly "thrush" or "thrash" (oral moniliasis) in children. The usual treatment is for the thrush doctor to blow three times in the child's mouth.[23;16;33;40;34;41] One Kentucky physician reports that it is "obvious" that the treatment works because of the natural course of the disease—to the believer, of course, it is just as obvious that the success is due to the power of the thrush doctor.[42] A variant appears in the classic *Pow-Wows or, The Long-Lost Friend*, first published in this country in 1820. The charm to banish whooping cough reads, "Cut three small bunches of hair from the crown of the head of a child that has never seen its father; sew this hair up in an unbleached rag and hang it around the neck of the child having the whooping cough. The thread with which the rag is sewed must also be unbleached."[43] This book is of particular interest because it is still available in a paperback edition and is widely disseminated. It is popular in the Pennsylvania Dutch country as well as in the South.[32;44] I obtained a copy in a candle-and-incense store in South Chicago where I was told that, together with an almanac, it was about all I needed to maintain health.

An instance of direct prenatal signaling is the child who is heard to cry three times in its mother's womb before birth; in Latin America this child will grow up to be a healer provided the mother tells no one.[45] One of my informants, a black woman, exhibited this trait *plus* she was the first child born after a set of twins, a belief found in West Africa and Haiti:[46]

> Some people say that I have the gift because I were born behind two twins. But I don't know, I always had that *urge* that I could cure anything! I've always felt like that. But my grandmother knew it *before* I were born. I cried three times in my mother's womb *before* I were born. Then she said, "That's the one. That's the one what's gonna be just exactly like me!" I was fortunate, I was born just exactly with the gift.[47]

In this instance the woman was literally programmed from birth as a healer and in fact began practice in childhood.

Twin births are not always viewed with pleasure, however. In the Ozarks they are associated with tragedy and misfortune, it may be said that twins "cannot be kept in bonds," or that the glance of a jealous twin can spoil the soup or kill pets[23;48;49] and houseplants. One old belief (19th century Sweden) combines several folk motifs. This is the belief that a "left twin" (one who survives a fellow twin) can cure thrush by blowing three times into the mouth of a patient of the opposite sex.[27]

The two commonest birth-associated statuses having to do with healing, however, are the Seventh Son or Seventh Sister and the child "born with the veil," or caul. The special power of the seventh son—ideally the seventh son of a seventh son—is attributed to a biblical passage. Shryock quotes an 1860 advertisement for a doctor who was a seventh son of a seventh daughter, was a seven-months child, walked at seven months and had moreover shed his teeth seven times![50] The seventh son or seventh sister is not restricted to healing just one illness but is more likely to be an all-round healer.[11;23;48;27;34;51]

The child born with a fragment of the amniotic membrane over the face is said to be born with the veil or caul. This centuries-old belief has also been found world-wide.[11;33;51;34] In some instances it is reported that the caul must be dried and saved or misfortune will befall the individual.[23;52] Like the seventh son or seventh sister the child born with the veil has more generalized powers and is often credited with second sight. Healers who advertise (under the rubric "Spiritual Advisors") in newspapers such as the Chicago *Defender* often cite being a seventh son or having been born with the veil as part of their credentials.[53] One woman reported that she was not only a seventh sister but that all seven of the siblings had been born with the veil; as the seventh, however, she possessed the most power. Again, most of these people are licensed ministers.

Folk curing techniques also vary widely. The methods of the bloodstopper, firedrawer and thrush doctor have already been mentioned. Those individuals who do a mail-order business usually ask the client to write or call to describe problems or symptoms and often respond by offering to burn candles, supplying an amulet or charm to be worn about the body plus the admonition to have faith in the healer and faith in God; the fee is usually at least twenty dollars and may be hundreds of dollars. It is always carefully explained that the money is *not* a charge but only a donation. (One woman who I consulted by mail instructed me to send nine straws from my broom. When I complied she informed me that "the Spirit" had told her that someone had cast not one but nine spells on me; each one, of course, would have to be removed separately. This would entail the burning of nine candles for each of the nine spells, the candles costing three dollars each). Such healers also often advertise that the patient need not even appear in person; the healer's power is so great that a cure can be sent by air.

Finally, I should like to discuss curing techniques described by three of my informants as they beautifully illustrate the wide disparity to be found in "faith healing." The first is much like the kind of thing that the public associates with the concept of the miracle cure. The setting is a healing revival in Miracle Valley, Arizona; the healer the evangelist whose "call" was described above; the patient a child with heart disease whose parents had brought her from another state in hope that she would be healed. The following excerpts illustrate two points, the contractual nature of the cure itself,.in which a bargain is made with God, and the fact that when Sister Erma is "anointed" she is not in perceptual control of surrounding events—she has to "shout 'till shout's gone." The very presence of the Holy Spirit, therefore, is the curing agent. The first speaker is the mother of the child:

> Well, it's gettin' close to the time for us to go home; my baby just won't get healed." I say, "Darlin', if God heal your baby, what would you do?" "Oh, I'd be the happiest soul!" I said, "In exchange, what would you do?" "Well, I would just be happy,". I said, "Would you give God the rest of your life to serve Him, cause you baby could die with this enlarged heart." She said, "Well, we're Episcopalians, we just come for the baby's healin'." So I said to her, "Darlin', probably you're holdin' back on the baby's healin'. God knows that this is all you want from Him. Many times this is why many people don't get healed, because they sittin' there and they want to snatch healin' like a hamburger and walk off with it. Like a hot dog stand or sumpin'. Well you have to give your life in exchange. God want you to promise Him sumpin'; you baby's life. Maybe He touched this child to get you to come to Him; He wants you to love Him."
>
> So this woman said, "Well, we just knew that our baby was gonna get healed tonight." I said, "Darlin', don't put God on the spot. You go runnin' like a hamburger, like a hot dog stand and get your baby healed, and then run back home. Maybe you need to feed on what they're feedin' down there from the pulpit; maybe you need to eat from that pulpit, there's somethin' good up there for you. That's why the Lord is keepin' you down here longer.". . . .
>
> Just about that time my hands went up and the Lord anointed me, and the power of God hit me and began to shout me all over the ground (this took place outside the church). And ever'body else *out* there, I mean, was shoutin'! And this little girl (the "baby") run to me and said, "Mama, Mama, I'm healed! I can feel that I don't have it no more!" And she (the mother) laid up on my shoulder and she said, "You don't know what you have done; you don't know what you have done!" But I'm just shoutin' away, I'm just gone in the Spirit. I just felt so good, I

couldn't stop. Somethin' about the Spirit of God, I can't stop shoutin' when I want to, I have to shout 'till shout's gone! So I looked around and he (the father) and I was shoutin' away. And the little girl had me by the skirt and was just a pullin' on me, and I was just a shoutin' away. He said, "Don't you know what you have done? Do you know what you have done?" Well, I thought I had did somethin', you know what I mean. I thought I'd hurt somebody or somethin'. Then I began to say to the Lord, "Lord, forgive me if I did anything wrong." But I was still shoutin' away. I didn't know what was happen cause I can't see, I close my eyes on the world, and then I'm gone away in the Spirit. So I looked around, and she say, "I'm healed, I'm healed!" I said, "Praise God!," and I looked around, everybody, that Spirit just went through ever'body; ever'body *down* there was shoutin'! Just like they was inside the church. The Spirit just cut through ever'body, and ever'body began to shout. . . .[8]

Sister Erma also gained added status because she succeeded in healing the child when the main evangelist had failed.

The healing techniques of Mother C., the woman who cried before birth and was the child born after a set of twins could not be more different. She maintains a "doctor's office" and holds regular office hours—patients who come to her wait their turn, sometimes sitting for hours in the waiting room. The average time spent with each person is twenty minutes but may be as long as an hour and a half. Mother C. sees herself as a "spiritual counselor" and is adept at ferreting out the problems of daily life which she feels are the basis for most of her clients problems:

. . .Like some of 'em says, I can't sleep, I can't sleep— Mother, why can't I sleep?" I'll sit there awhile, talk around, kid around with 'em, then I tell them they're *sick*, they're thinkin' too hard about somethin'. Their bills are worryin' them. You know how times is now, things is changed'. 'n everything is so high. Some people get such a small wage, don't make much money. They can't make ends meet. And then it *come* to them when they stop still, like they'll lie down and get to thinkin'. It gets into the mind, they's so weak they can't throw it off. Well, next thing you know it's daylight!. . .

. . .Some buys too much, go downtown cause they can get things on the credit. Well, they over*do* it! See, they get more than they can *pay* for! Then when the time come for

them to pay for what they got, they don't see no way out
of it! They don't want to lose what they *have*—nobody
does. "Where is I gonna get the money to pay this and
that. . ." and the next thing, he *sick*! I get a lot of people
like that. But they don't know what's wrong with 'em, no,
they don't! They doesn't, that's why they hunt somebody
to advise 'em, or counsel with them, you know. I get
people like that ever' day. Well, I just tell people the
truth, you know, and it's *right.* You can look at your
budget, what you got comin' in. And then, go accordin'
. . . .The most sickness there is, I think, is *nerves!*
Every'body I see is nervous! Just *tense* nervous, you know?
They get to thinkin', then they get a headache, and from
that go to vomiting. Cause they stirred up that nerve in the
stomach. I see a lot of people like that, comin' to me all
the time. They say, "Well, I went to the doctor, and they
took a x-ray. They couldn't find nothin'! They say nothin's
wrong with me! They say I'm nervous, but I hurt here,
and I hurt there." And I say, "No wonder, you *are* nervous.
I wouldn't say you not nervous. True. You *made* yourself
like that.[47]

The following passage illustrates clearly that, unlike Sister
Erma, she is in full control of the situation and directly
manipulates the doctor/patient relationship:

I talk to people and I get them to thinkin'. I talk to
people and *watch* them, seein' is it takin' effect. And it *is,*
then I pour it on! Cause that's what I want, you know, I
want them to believe what I'm sayin'. And then when they
do, I pour it on, see. Then they get so *strong!* See, they
gainin' all the time when I'm counselin' to 'em. All of it is
on the mind, bad thoughts. Whatever you *think,* well,
that's what you are. So many people don't know about
life, they stumble and blunders. I feel sorry for 'em, they
in the dark. They don't have no confidence, no faith in
their*self!* You have to *first* place faith in yourself, *believe*
that you can do a thing. If you get enough faith in *yourself,*
then you can face *anything.* I don't care *what* it is, you can
face it. But if you don't have no faith in yourself, and
waver, well, you can't make it stick. . . .

Now, that's one thing that I love, too, to make people
happy. I go all out the way to make someone happy. You
know, feel good. Come to me cryin', in tears, ever'thing,
then I think right quick: What can I do to make them
smile? Then I'll go all out, and they'll smile. I don't care
how burdened down, next thing you know we'll have a big
conversation, and laughin' up a breeze! And that's my

> desire too, that's what I do, ever' day of my life. When they come to me, ever' day, they leave laughin'. I don't care how heartbroken they are, how sorry, what feelin' bad they were. They go out feelin' good.[47]

The final example is one which, like the healing of the "polio" which opened this essay, shows the *collective* power of the community. That is, no one individual has enough power to heal but banded together they can even raise the newly dead. The following example differs from the other two as well in that the patient does not come to healing services willingly—although her "illness" is presented as alcoholism it is clear that she has deviated from the acceptable norms of the group in other ways as well:

> I have seen alcoholics, I've seen an alcoholic cured, a female. In my home town. Came to the church, she was drunk, she was the biggest rip in the town, one of the biggest! I don't know how many babies she *had* had, you know, just [had], and she didn't take care of 'em, she was always runnin' constantly, and her mother was a good old Christian woman. Finally it got to the source she was always seein' bugs and snakes, she was really *soused!* And her mother brought her into the church cryin' and beggin' help for her. And she bent her down there and first they prayed away the *drunk*, the stupor she was in, the bugs and all the things she was fightin' and seein', they prayed *that* away. They prayed the Devil out. Then they started a course of prayin' for her soul, all of this stuff to leave her body and to place her in God's hands, watch over her and touch her. And she jerked and pulled and there was all kinds of friction there on that floor! They wrestled with her and everything! I mean there was *somethin'* takin' hold, I don't know what it was. There was a lot of church members there and she laid there and jerked and pulled and fought with them 'til every one of 'em was sweatin'! It was hours later, and I stayed for the whole thing, I watched it. And that woman was sober when she got up offen that floor. And the next night she was at church and from then on she was a good christian woman.[1]

The community judged her, the community healed her, the community reintegrated her into full membership.

As might be expected, the failure for a cure to take place is also viewed in a relogous context. Sometimes, of course, it is not meant to be, ". . .the Lord don't intend to heal 'em all. . .it ain't His will."[54] Mother C. says that if a patient is not healed it is not *her* fault it is because they didn't have enough faith. And, since healing is on a contractual basis with the Almighty, breach-of-contract is mortally dangerous. A backslid sinner is flirting with disaster:

> I have knowed of bringing the dead to life. You can't be dead *long*. I have never done it but the church did. This takes more than one person. Actually, it takes a party of people to be together at the sime, say, a baby died. Now, my aunt's baby died once. But she made a promise, that's the way I understood it. I've heard of it happenin' before. She made a promise to the Lord, if He let her baby lived she wouldn't ever cuss again, use His name in vain, she would go to church and become a Christian and live for *Him*. Just to let her baby live. Well, she prayed too, see, and she made these promises, these vows, right at the time. It lived, but it only lived a month, two months. She went back on *her* word. It died. It took pneumonia, then, and it died within three hours. She thought it was because she broke her vow.[1]

For any misfortune, in fact, as the spiritual goes, The Failure's Not in God It's in Me: "I haven't done all that I should...must be something wrong I have done...If I lose my soul because I did not give God control...the failure is not in God, it's in me."[17] If such judgments seem harsh it is imperative to see them in social and cultural context. Belief in supernatural external control of events may make the individual seem passive, dependent and fatalistic to the science and action-oriented health professional but viewing patients holding such views as of sub-normal intelligence is of utility to neither party. Instead, it is more useful to inquire into the life experiences which require the individual to seek such explanations for problems in living. Sister Erma, that is, can say

> I got joy, I got peace, I got ever'thing I want. There's nobody no happier than I am. I don't have no childrens, I don't have no husband, I have Jesus. He's childrens, He's husband, He's *ever'thing!* He's a great consolation to me. I'm not in no good-lookin' house, but inside I'm just as rich and happy as anybody else. I don't know nobody no happier than I am. I don't have luxury and all, but I have a home up yonder. This home, I'm not bothered about nothin' here, I'm lookin' beyond. I'm lookin' to meet the Lord on a cloud, on that resurrection morin'.[8]

She may indeed have joy and she may have peace. She also has diabetes mellitus, hypertension and arthritis and lives in a state which voted down Medicaid. At the time of the interviews (1971) her total income was $118/month, although she was adjudged totally disabled and unable to work. Instead of puzzling over the mental or emotional state which allows Sister Erma and others like her to talk to God we might puzzle over the system which allows so many people to live under the conditions where God seems to be the only listener. Instead of wondering that people can believe that a man-who-has-never-seen-his-father can cure oral moniliasis by blowing three times into an infant's mouth we might wonder at the socio-environmental conditions which allow such infections to flourish among poor children.

The preceding pages have described how life events both large and small tend to be fitted into a religious framework for many poor rural Southerners both white and black. It *is* a framework that reinforces feelings of helplessness, of insignificance, of being at the mercy of powerful external forces. Magic and religion do entertwine in the attempt to solve the problems of everyday living and such attempts are too often seen as ignorance, as superstition, as evidence of subnormal mentality when they come to the attention of the health professional. And, as the problem is seen as being one of ignorance, the answer is often seen in terms of "education": and the education in question has to do with weaning the patient away from the use of home remedies and patented medicines, with eliminating the "quack" healer, with presenting "real" medicine as so patently superior that presentation is all that is required for instant acceptance. This viewpoint is not only naive but, in medical parlance, treats the symptom not the disease.

The informants among whom I work *may* be ignorant and poorly educated but they are not stupid; there are some things that they know and know well. They know, for instance, that they do not share fully in the social/economic pie. They know that many of their most valued and deeply held beliefs are different from those of the mainstream middle-class citizen, and these same beliefs are seen as laughable and ridiculous. They are quite aware that some of their medical beliefs and practices are not shared by main-stream medicine and they largely know which beliefs these are: this does not result in their being dropped, it results in their being hidden. Too many poor patients are also quite aware that many physicians and ancillary health workers see them as shiftless, dirty, ignorant, lazy and inferior and would prefer not to have to deal with them. In most cases individuals do *not* select unorthodox healers because they do not see the advantages of going to a "real" doctor; they have probably already been to one. I believe, in fact, that the people I have been talking about would use modern medicine almost exclusively if it were truly available to them on acceptable terms—in too many cases the "witch doctor" exists *because* of the medical profession, not in spite of it. The bloodstopper, the firedrawer, the thrush doctor, the faith healer are all extant because they meet felt needs in a portion of the population who would otherwise be largely unserviced healthwise. But the individual who believes in the power of the seventh son can also say

> I believe in doctors. There was doctors here when Jesus was here; the doctors are here for a purpose. [They have] a knowledge; I'll say in a word, a gift. People have these gifts. You put these gifts in practice and they can do these things. It's from God.[8]

Unfortunately, it may be easier for her to find a seventh son than a physician willing to take her as a patient.

The description of the medical beliefs of any group, however interesting, is not enough if needed changes are to be made in the delivery of health care. It is perhaps too easy for the anthropologist in a medical school setting to serve only as a cultural interpreter, to be the person responsible for bringing differences in the perception of health and illness within a population to the attention of future physicians, in explaining why such differences occur and in making suggestions as to how modern medical care can best be offered so as to be acceptable to a clientele which might differ in socio-cultural background from that of the deliverers of such care.

In the clinical setting, however, it has to be decided whether to present a modern treatment in an old form to make it more palatable to the patient, and, if this is to be done, how it is to be done without compromising the standards of the physician. Here again the anthropologist can give opinions as to the probable acceptability of a particular treatment regimen or even how to couch it so that it will "fit" a particular cultural pattern without having to make the ethical decisions incumbent on the practitioner. In point of fact if the anthropologist is well acquainted with the belief system of the client population it should be relatively easy to frame many treatment regimens into cultural terms understandable to the patient. No one, of course, would recommend something which is in direct conflict with cultural values and therefore almost certain to be rejected. On the other hand, should a health professional couch medical advice in a way which is acceptable to the patient but which violates what he or she believes to be true? And when is it essential to correct misinformation and when does it not matter? Often the severity of the problem seems to be the most decisive factor—the use of home remedies for *minor* health problems may be ignored, for example, but deplored as dangerous and stupid when people use home remedies for more serious illnesses. What this implies is that *we* will decide what bits of cultural health baggage are to be kept, *we* will decide which are dangerous and which are merely quaint. But the simple contains the complex and the view which allows the "harmless" home remedy by logical extension allows the dangerous: gargling hot salt water for a sore throat may be harmless; drinking turpentine in an attempt to induce abortion is not. The decision to let patients keep old-fashioned but harmless practices, therefore, also allows the retention of potentially lethal ones.

The decision to interact with folk healers in health care delivery involves a number of issues above and beyond whether they should be allowed to exist. They *do* exist. They *do* fulfill expectations of the role of the healer in the minds of many. In some cases it must be recognized that only a certain kind of healer is believable to deal with some problems. In many instances therefore the folk healer *is* the specialist of choice, when he or she is better able to understand and to appropriately handle certain difficulties. It is therefore important to recognize the presence of folk healers in the community, to know what problems they are adept at solving, to know when it might be appropriate to make a referral to such a healer and when not, and to make efforts to understand what influences the selection of a healer—professional or folk—by individuals in the population to be served.

It is equally important to realize that a blanket decision to give official sanction to folk healers is more romantic than realistic and may not in the long run be of service to the healer, to the patient, or to the medical profession. As one example consider the kinds of problems which might arise by bringing the "born" healer into the clinical setting. Individuals who have been thought special—and specially treated—since birth may have a great deal of charisma. Mother C. is such a person and her own medical practice illustrates some of the considerations which must be taken into account. There is no doubt that she performs a valuable service as a "spiritual counselor;" that does *not* mean, as she also contends, that she can cure *any* illness by laying on hands. She also exemplifies a potential trouble area in that she is believed to have the power to cure illnesses caused by witchcraft. This is a prime example of the folk illness thought not amenable to modern medical treatment so that a special healer must be sought out. There is abundant evidence that the individual who believes in witchcraft may become seriously ill at the suspicion of a spell or hex.[55-58] Given the belief that it *is* possible and that the physician *cannot* help, this makes the presence of a healer who can remove the charm essential: for this reason some physicians have learned to refer patients to such healers when necessary.[59] There is an equally compelling reason for such individuals to *not* be brought into the health center, however, and this is that they may be considered able to do harm as well as good—that they may have the power to "put on" a hex as well as take it off. The individual may therefore be greatly feared and might keep away as many people as they attracted to the health facility. It needs to be carefully thought out, therefore, before offering office space to someone who may have the reputation of being able to kill with magic as well as heal.

Again the basic problem remains the same: we are

treating the symptom not the cause. What needs to be changed is the system which allows people to live in a social setting so hostile and threatening that they would be foolish *not* to believe in externalized evil. In the short run, therefore, we need to be able to recognize folk illnesses and call in folk healers when appropriate, or to refer our patients to them. In the long run, however, what is needed is a restructuring of American society so that unorthodox healers are no longer required and so that people like Sister Erma really *do* "have ever'thing!"

NOTES

[1]From taped interview with 29 year old white woman raised in West Virginia, now residing in Michigan, March, 1975.

[2]Frank, Jerome D.: *Persuasion and Healing, A Comparative Study of Psychotherapy.* (revised edition 1973) The Johns Hopkins University Press, Baltimore, 1961, p. 76.

[3]Torrey, E. Fuller: *The Mind Game: Witchdoctors and Psychiatrists.* Emerson Hall Publishers, New York, 1972.

[4]Personal communication from physician, Lansing, Michigan, April 1975.

[5]King, Lester S. (editor): *A History of Medicine.* Penguin Books Ltd., Harmondsworth, England, 1971, p. 54.

[6]Rose, Louis: *Faith Healing.* Revised edition, Penguin Books Ltd., Harmondsworth, England, 1971, p. 175.

[7]Nolen, William A.: *Healing: A Doctor in Search of a Miracle.* Random House, New York 1974.

[8]Snow, Loudell F.: "The Sun Don't Shine No Way All the Time": Popular Medicine in a Black Neighborhood. In *Ethnic Medicine in the Southwest,* Edward H. Spicer, editor, University of Arizona Press, Tucson, 1975, in press.

[9]Snow, Loudell F.: *The Medical System of a Group of Urban Blacks.* Unpublished doctoral dissertation, University of Arizona, Tucson 1971. A current research project involves comparing beliefs and attitudes concerning female reproduction of women from four ethnic groups in Michigan, including both black and Southern white informants: 1975.

[10]Dorson, Richard: *American Folklore.* University of Chicago Press, Chicago, 1959, pp. 90-91; 100.

[11]Emrich, Duncan: *Folklore on the American Land.* Little, Brown and Company, Boston, 1972, pp. 613; 610; 637.

[12]Pearsal, Marion: "Healthways in a Mountain County." *Mountain Life and Work* 36:4:7-13, 1960.

[13]Wiener, Jack: "Mental Health Highlights." *American Journal of Orthopsychiatry* 39:3:530-531, 1969.

[14]Pearsall, Marion: *Little Smoky Ridge.* University of Alabama Press, Birminghan, 1959.

[15]Persall, Marion: "Some Behavioral Factors in the Control of Tuberculosis in a Rural County." *American Review of Respiratory Disease* 85:200-210, 1962.

[16]Murphree, Alice H.: "A Functional Analysis of Southern Folk Beliefs concerning Birth." *American Journal of Obstetrics and Gynecology* 102:125-134, 1968.

[17]Simpson, Robert B.: *A Black Church: Ecstasy in a World of Trouble.* Unpublished doctoral dissertation, Washington University, St. Louis, pp. 64; 7, 1970.

[18]Bourguignon, Erika E.: "Afro-American Religions: Traditions and Transformations." In *Black America*, John Szwed, editor, Basic Books, New York, 1970.

[19]Clark, Kenneth B.: *Dark Ghetto. Dilemmas of Social Power.* Harper Torchbooks (1967), Harper & Row, New York, pp. 174-175, 1965.

[20]Gaver, Jessyca Russell: *Pentecostalism.* Award Books, Universal Publishing and Distributing Corporation, New York, 1971.

[21]Fauset, Arthur Huff: *Black Gods of the Metropolis.* University of Pennsylvania Press, Philadelphia, 1944.

[22]*Holy Bible.* Book of Genesis 1:29; cf. also Ezekiel 47:12; Revelations 22:2.

[23]Randolph, Vance: *Ozark Superstitions.* Columbia University Press, New York, pp. 93; 123; 136-137; 203; 207, 1947.

[24]Morton, Julia F.: *Folk Remedies of the Low Country.* E. A. Seemann Publishing, Inc., Miami, 1974.

[25]Murphree, Alice H., and Mark V. Barrow: "Physician Dependence, Self-Treatment Practices, and Folk Remedies in a Rural Area." *Southern Medical Journal* 63:403-408, 1970.

[26]Fabrega, Horacio, Jr., and Daniel B. Silver: *Illness and Shamanistic Curing in Zinacantan.* Stanford University Press, Stanford, p. 31, 1973.

[27]Black, William George: *Folk Medicine; A Chapter in the History of Culture.* Elliot Stock, Publisher, London, 1883, pp. 76-77; 136-138.

[28]Wigginton, Eliot (editor): *The Foxfire Book.* Doubleday & Company, Garden City, New York, 1972, pp. 346-368.

[29]Cooper, Horton: *North Carolina Mountain Folklore and Miscellany.* Johnson Publishing Co., Murfreeboro, N.C., 1972, p. 77.

[30]Dorson, Richard: *Bloodstoppers and Bearwalkers.* Harvard University Press, Cambridge, 1956, p. 150.

[31]Dorson, Richard: *Buying the Wind. Regional Folklore in the United States.* University of Chicago Press, Chicago, 1964, p. 115.

[32]Jones, Louis C.: "Practitioners of Folk Medicine." *Bulletin of the History of Medicine* 23:480-493, 1949.

[33]Dorson, Richard: *American Negro Folktales.* Fawcett Publi-

cations, Inc., Greenwich, Conn., 1956, pp. 211-212; 282.

34Stekert, Ellen: "Focus for Conflict: Southern Medical Beliefs in Detroit." In *The Urban Experience and Folk Tradition*. A. Paredes and E. Stekert, editors, University of Texas Press, Austin, 1971, pp. 95-127.

35Snow, Loudell F.: "Folk Medical Beliefs and Their Implications for Care of Patients." *Annals of Internal Medicine* 81:82-96, 1974.

36Alland, Alexander: "Possession in a Revivalist Negro Church." *Journal for the Scientific Study of Religion* 1:2-12, 1961.

37Sussex, James N., and Hazel Weidman: "Some Dynamic and Functional Characteristics of a Culture-Bound Syndrome in Urban USA: Falling-Out in Miami." Paper presented at the 72nd Annual Meeting of the American Anthropological Association, New Orleans, La., 1973.

38Ludwig, Arnold: Altered States of Consciousness. In *Trance and Possession States*. Raymond Prince, editor, R. M. Bucke Memorial Society, Montreal, pp. 69-95, 1968.

39Kahn, Kathy: *Hillbilly Women*. Doubleday Company, Garden City, New York, 1973, pp. 141-142.

40Cameron, Vivian Knowles: *Folk Beliefs Pertaining to Health of the Southern Negro*. Unpublished Master's thesis, Northwestern University, Evanston, 1930, p. 29.

41Webb, Julie Yvonne: "Louisiana Voodoo and Superstitions Related to Health." *HSMHA Health Reports* 86:4:291-301, 1971.

42Hughes, Walter T.: "Superstitions and Home Remedies Encountered in Present-Day Pediatric Practice in the South." *Journal of the Kentucky State Medical Association* 61:25-27, 1963.

43Hohman, John George: *Pow-Wows, or, The Long-Lost Friend. A Collection of Mysterious Arts and Remedies for Man as well as Animals*. Published for the trade (no re-publication date), p. 15, 1820.

44Powdermaker, Hortense: *After Freedom*. The Viking Press, New York, 1939, p. 295.

45Foster, George M.: "Relationships between Spanish and Spanish-American Folk Medicine." *Journal of American Folklore* 66:201-217, 1953.

46Metraux, Alfred: *Voodoo in Haiti*. Oxford University Press, New York, 1959, p. 146.

47Snow, Loudell F.: "I was Born Just Exactly with the Gift." An Interview with a Voodoo Practitioner. *Journal of American Folklore* 86:272-281, 1973.

48Parsons, Elsie Clews: "Folk-Lore of the Sea Islands, South Carolina." *American Folk-Lore Society Memoirs* XVI, Cambridge, 1923 pp. 197-198.

49Kay, Margarita: *Health and Illness in the Barrio: Women's Point of View*. Unpublished doctoral dissertation, University of Arizona, Tucson, 1972, p. 146.

50Shryock, Richard Harrison: Medical Practice in the Old South. In *Medicine in America: Historical Essays*. The Johns Hopkins Press, Baltimore, 1966, pp. 49-70?

[51]Hand, Wayland D. (editor): Popular Beliefs and Superstitions from North Carolina. Volume VI of the *Frank C. Brown Collection of North Carolina Folklore*. Duke University Press, Durham, 1961, pp. 3-68.

[52]Forbes, Thomas Rogers: *The Midwife and the Witch*. Yale University Press, Cambridge, 1966, pp. 95-97.

[53]Snow, Loudell F.: Mail Order Preventions and Cures for Witchcraft. Paper presented at the 72nd Annual Meeting of the American Anthropological Association, New Orleans, La., 1973.

[54]Withers, Carl: The Folklore of a Small Town. In *Medical Care*. W. Richard Scott and Edmund Volkart, editors, John Wiley & Sons, Inc., New York, 1966, pp. 233-246.

[55]Tinling, David C.: "Voodoo, Root Work, and Medicine." *Psychosomatic Medicine* 29:483-490, 1967.

[56]Spell, John E.: "Hypnosis in the Treatment of the 'Hexed' Patient." *American Journal of Psychiatry* 124:3:311-316, 1967.

[57]Wintrob, Ronald: Hexes, Roots, Snake Eggs? MD. vs. Occult. *Medical Opinion* 1:7:55-61, 1972.

[58]Clinicopathologic Conference: Case Presentation (BCH No. 469861). *Johns Hopkins Medical Journal* 120:186-199, 1967.

[59]Wintrob, Ronald: "The Influence of Others: Witchcraft and Rootword as Explanations of Behavior Disturbances." *Journal of Nervous and Mental Disease* 156:318-326, 1973.

TRADITIONAL HEALING AND THE NEW HEALTH CENTER IN ETHIOPIA*

Simon D. Messing, Ph.D.

When rural health centers are established in "Third World" independent countries, the modern-trained, indigenous health officers and their staff frequently hold what may be called "sub-colonial attitudes" toward traditional types of healers. The modern training has emphasized errors of diagnosis and treatment of the old-time, rural pragmatist, and has frequently created unbounded admiration in the minds of the new health officers and their staff for anti-biotic "miracle drugs" and the superiority of modern psychiatry over the "medicine man" or "witch doctor." Even health officers not overwhelmingly imbued with their own superiority wonder whether it is appropriate for them to collaborate with local healers whose practices they define as "backward" or "magical." Sometimes the health officer even avoids being seen in public conversing with such a healer, for fear that this may augment the healer's practice.

Traditional healers, on their part, frequently desire such collaboration, in order to improve their methods. In return, they offer the trust in which the local population holds them, which could be very useful to the health officer to make his patients comfortable, and to promote the preventive and sanitary changes which are supposed to constitute his major task.

Such confrontations were observed in rural Ethiopia during the 1960's under the auspices of USAID-Public Health field studies. This agency had largely sponsored the training of Health Officers and was proceeding to supervision of their work in a variety of ecological and ethnic regions of the country. The new Health Center mentioned here was being established in the small town of Hosaina, district of Kam-

---

*The original version of this article was prepared as a paper for the symposium organized by Dr. P. Singer on "Western Medical Practices and Indigenous Healers," at the meeting of the Society for Applied Anthropology at Montreal, April 5-9, 1972.

batta, in southwest Ethiopia. In this region the indigenous Kambatta-Gudela population had been conquered by the dominant Amhara ethnic group in the late 19th century. Since the conquerors had arrived with rifles, their descendants who settled and married local women and who still occupy upper social status are referred to as *neftenya lij* meaning "sons of guns." During the study, Hosaina had only a dry-weather road to the capital of Addis Ababa, but heavy trucks maintained trade from the local market most of the year. The local majority officially adheres to the Coptic-Christian ("Orthodox") Church of Ethiopia, and a minority to Islam, but in the surrounding countryside many older religious beliefs and practices are retained. In Hosaina town modern facilities include an elementary school, truck and landrover transport, flour mills, a hotel-bar, private electricity. Some of the owners of these enterprises serve on the health council.

In its demographic pattern the town also differs from the nearby countryside. Among the residents of the town's 4000 persons, 36% of the heads of households consist of women abandoned by their husbands. Most eke out a living as "beer-brewers at home," with the younger and more attractive ones augmenting this income as prostitutes. Another poor element in the local population consists of aged widows living alone in huts on the outskirts of town. A number of these women had been taken from homes in distant ethnic regions of the Wollamo, Galla, Agaw and other tribes during their childhood, in the time of slavery. They had lost contact with their families and even forgotten their ancestral languages. One of these recalled that as a little girl she had given water to the wounded after the Battle of Koram (1909) and had been taken into slavery shortly thereafter.

The chief function of the little town is to serve as "Saturday market" for huge crowds of peasants, and as business center for traders, both retail and wholesale. Most peasants are sharecroppers, and in dry years their crops of maize, cabbage and so on are so small that survival is a problem after paying the rent that can be as high as 4/5 of the produce. Poor townspeople sometimes suffer when traders create artificial shortages of cereals by transporting regional produce to distant markets like Addis Ababa, where higher prices can be obtained, thus increasing the local cost of living. One trade item of health interest is soap. When business is slow, some traders add a free sewing needle to each bar of soap purchased. During the study, the private electricity was operating for only four hours each evening in the center of town, and even then it ceased when the kerosene fuel supply diminished. Thus the health center could not rely on electricity.

This was the culture scene in existence when the Health Officer arrived to introduce modern health practices *and* training had not included awareness that he was not starting from a *tabula rasa*. The medical vacuum had long been filled by indigenous healers within the limitations of their knowledge and resources.

Indigenous Healers: Status and Practices

The two chief indigenous healers in the town differed not only in sex, but also in social status and types of practice. Thus, they were not in competition. One was a male aged about 50, an Amhara from what constituted the local upper class, i.e. of *neftenya lij* ancestry. He claimed that he derived more income from his own land and coffee trees than from his own sons. He was illiterate, but had sent one son to Addis Ababa where he succeeded in reaching the 9th grade in school.

This healer's establishment was on a pleasant, grassy meadow about half an hour's walking distance east of the town, where he and his sons occupied several well-built huts typical of small, fief-holding farmers. He claimed that he had drifted into the practice of healing gradually. The only method he had learned from his father was first aid, particularly the setting of broken bones. Then he began having many children and paying fees to other *woggesha* (healers). He observed their practices and experimented with them. Soon neighbors addressed him as *hakim* (the honorific address for any healer), and asked his help as a favor. His reputation greatly expanded when he cured the daughter of the local large landowner who held the title *Gerazmatch*

54

(roughly:baron). The six-months-old baby had swallowed an empty pistol cartridge. Taken to the nearest Mission hospital for X-rays, the foreign doctor recommended that the baby be sent to Addis Ababa for surgery. The father refused and consulted the *woggesha*, who toasted a cabbage leaf until soft, rolled it to a point, pushed it down the baby's throat and pulled. There was some bleeding, the baby fainted, was awakened, and given some water and a traditional herbal laxative. Several days later the cartridge emerged in the stool. After this event and the reward he received, he began to practice regularly, charging fees.

A common practice of his, widespread in Ethiopia, is the cutting out of the uvula, the central part of the upper soft palate. The uvula is blamed for many respiratory ailments, especially in children. When operating on infants, he uses a snare made of two strands of twisted horsehair. In case of adults he employs a fine wire. Another traditional and common operation is performed when a child grows poorly and suffers from diarrhea. In this case he examines the gums and extracts the root of a budding tooth with one of the two screwdrivers he carries at all times. He is also famous for treating hemmorhoids with a shrinking compound made of herbs and butter. In severe cases he cauterizes the piles by burning them with one of nine different types of twigs. Internal body ailments are sometimes treated by burning the nearest skin surface. He treats eye infections by vertical cuts of the eyebrows, so that the blood will wash out the disease as it flows over the eyeball.

A frequent practice of his is circumcision of males, and, more rarely, the cutting out of the clitoris of girls. The age of male clients for this operation ranges from seven to eight days, in case of religious Copts, to men of 30 from among the local Gudela ethnic group. The latter are the original "pagan" inhabitants of this region who come to him for this operation when they wish to be accepted by the Coptic Christians for intermarriage. The local Coptic clergy requires the operation as proof of sincerity from "pagan" converts. For a similar reason girls are brought to him for clitoridectomy at age 12-13, as a preliminary to marriage to a Copt, although this is an unusually late age for this operation in Ethiopia. In order to reduce bleeding and swelling, the healer applies a wet leaf and uses a vein of the leaf to tie a bandage.

He is also consulted when childbirth complications occur, such as breech births or a retained placenta. It is in such obstetrical cases that the Health Officer most frequently encounters him. Like most traditional healers, he concocts his own ointments. Wheat powder is used as a ingredient against skin infections, wounds, and scabies; he uses it on humans, mules, donkeys, and horses. His fees charged for such routine treatments range from 12 cents - 40 cents for poor clients, to $1.25 for what are locally considered rich clients. When mixing powders against serious ailments such as paralysis of infants (blamed on spiritual infection from certain birds), he also pronounces a verbal formula which he memorized by listening to his wife's brother, a literate astrologer, who had once been a church student. But otherwise he does not employ spirit-healing. Instead he refers epileptics and mental patients (diagnosed as possibly *zar*— "possessed") to *zar* doctors on the plateau (Amhara) or to *Qalitcha* spirit healers in the lowlands of the Galla ethnic group. It is possible that he splits fees in this case, but he does not admit this.

It is typical of this man, and other herbologist-surgeons (*Woggesha*), that they take a pragmatic attitude to methods of treatment. He is interested in observing modern medicine. For dental surgery he has added a pair of pliers to the kit of uvula-cutter and screwdrivers he carries with him. His most common cases now are fractures, including compound fractures, "gland trouble," and retained placentas and other birth complications, for the treatment of which he is continuously improving his lubricants.

The best-known female healer in the locality is an old woman of a black physical type which was viewed by local people as indicative of former slave status, of Shanqalla (Sudanese border tribe) ancestry. She admitted that she had been brought to the region in childhood, but claimed Gala ethnic ancestry—somewhat higher social status. Her husband was an aged Amhara peasant, but not a landowner; he always stood by her side during interviews. Actually she did not need this support of a higher-status person, for she clearly dominated the situation. Though barefoot, poorly dressed, and inhabiting a simple, round hut (*tuqul*) half an hour's walking distance west of town, no trace of servility remained from her former slave status, and she displayed a calm, self-assured manner that inspired confidence and was probably her chief stock-in-trade.

She did, however, frequently emphasize her adherence to Coptic Christian (Amhara) beliefs and attitudes. Thus, she explained her entry into the practice of healing on the grounds that "God has taught me how to help pregnant women," to which she had gradually added further procedures. She was often consulted on complications relating to delivery, and also did abdominal massage for many ailments, including "rupture." She denied cutting the uvula, but she approved of the practice, referring clients in need of this operation to healers of the Guadela ethnic farmers or to ironsmiths of the Fuga caste of the Galla ethnic group. Female circumcision, particularly clitoridectomy, made up a considerable part of her practice. The age range of girls undergoing the operation ranged from seven days to 15 years, depending on their ethnic group. Prior to the operation she purged the patient's intestines with the herbal laxative from the *Kosso* (Quassia) tree, for sanitary reasons and to reduce bleeding. *Kosso* was also an ingredient of the poultice, made with butter and certain leaves, and applied to cover the wound. Illiterate and untrained in Coptic theology, she nevertheless insisted that "the Virgin Mary does not want a female to sleep with a man unless she has been operated on properly." An additional reason she gave for urging the operation was also typical of the Amhara. They believe that a non-operated girl would be over-sexed, hence unfaithful to her husband, or so tense from sexual frustration that she would break all the dishes in the home. She was so sure of these facts that she retorted to the interviewer: "Don't you circumcise your girls?" Convalescence for 15-year old girls ranged from 3 to 8 days, during which they were fed butter and other "good" foods. Her fees ranged from as little as 8 cents charged poor people, to $1.25 charged the "local rich" for the same services.

While she does not practice any spiritual healing, she treats her medicines with the respect reserved for sacred objects. When she carries a medicine and someone speaks to her, she places it on the ground before answering, lest the spirit of the plant be offended or ritually contaminated. One of the more common recent additions to her practice were "yellow jaundice" cases (probably hepatitis). For this she prescribes a special leaf which patients would chew and swallow.

Like most people in the little town, she was aware of the miraculous effect of the hypodermic needle filled with antibiotics. But this was expensive on the open market and she therefore recommended it only in special cases. For example, when called upon to perform a circumcision on a child of parents who were both *wurde*, chronic syphilitics, she would postpone the operation until the child reached the age of 7 or 8 years, and administer an antibiotic injection following the operation in order to prevent complications.

The indigenous healers therefore are not exploiters. They fill the medical vacuum as best they can, and stand ready as possible agents for improvements.

The practices of such traditional healers raises two questions in the minds of modern health promoters:

(1) The problem of those traditional procedures that are obviously harmful. In the above-mentioned examples, the cutting of the uvula and clitoridectomy carry unnecessary risks of infection. Moreover, the former operation does not cure what it is intended to cure, and the latter operation is psychologically harmful in the view of modern medicine. Are the healers therefore to be regarded as exploiters of their ignorant patients, like quacks at a carnival? It would seem unjust to levy that accusation. The traditional healers fill the medical vacuum as best they know, are eager to improve their methods, and many of them stand ready to be trained as possible agents of medical change—perhaps of the "bare-foot doctor" or "feldsher" variety.

(2) The failure to fill the "medical vacuum" more rapidly by modern medicine requires an explanation. At first glance it would seem to constitute a failure on the part of the present governments of the developing regions. In

Ethiopia, the attempt to meet this challenge was made by developing "generalized, decentralized, preventive" Health Centers to serve the rural regions.

The Health Center and Indigenous Responses

Due to the severe shortage of modern medical personnel in Ethiopia, the Public Health College was founded in the provincial town of Gondar, in 1954, to train paramedical personnel. Since contagious disease is the greatest medical problem in Ethiopia, and therefore preventable, the concepts of prevention and decentralization were emphasized in the Public Health College. This approach also promised greater productive results for the economic input. The original sponsorship was largely with American funds, and three categories were to be trained. High school graduates were recruited for the top category, that of Health Officer, who thereupon underwent three years of training plus one year of supervision. He was expected to supervise preventive procedures including immunizations and public health, and also conduct a first-aid clinic. Since most of them had been recruited from what might be called an upper-middle class, life in small towns like Hosaina presented a hardship for them, and as soon as a medical school for physicians opened in Addis Ababa most of them opted for that after a few years of rural service. The second category, called Community Nurse, was recruited from girls who usually had at least a 10th grade education. They were given two years of training plus one of supervision, and expected to conduct mother-and-child services including home visits. Most married after a few years of service, in some cases a Health Officer, so that their training was not entirely lost. The third category, called Sanitarian, was recruited mostly from graduates of elementary schools, often from what might be called lower-middle or upper-lower socio-economic levels which could not provide any other professional careers. His one-year training and one-year supervision provided basic hygiene and health education lessons. He was expected to attempt to break the cycle of re-infection from human waste to food, as in dysentery, and other insect-borne and water-borne diseases. In addition to supervising the Community Nurse and Sanitarian, the Health Officer also had the task of supervising a 4th, pre-existing category, that of the "dresser." As the name implies, this dresser of wounds had received informal training as hospital orderly, sometimes in wartime. His work included simple first aid, wielding the hypodermic needle and general assistance in the clinic, but he was also available for assignment to a wider circle of villages which lacked any modern health facility. Since transportation difficulties in the hinterland required travel by mule or on foot, supervision of village dressers was bound to be minimal.

Our fieldwork showed that people on communities all over Ethiopia regarded the health officer and his staff as an additional sort of *hakim* (healer), and that they expected him to abandon his schedule of teaching prevention the moment a clinical need arose. Most insistent were the local officials, who regarded him as their personal physician for home calls and also for all their relatives, friends and retainers. People usually treated the community nurse as another type of midwife, and if she herself had not had a baby, her instructions were merely listened to politely but regarded as theoretical and not followed. The sanitarian found least acceptance of all, for there was not traditional precedent for his role. When he urged the digging of latrines or warned butchers to screen their meat from flies, he was usually regarded as a nuisance.

The health officer had encountered the following diseases in the Hosaina clinic: Intestinal ailments (esp. roundworm), infectious hepatitis, eye infections (trachoma and conjunctivitis), venereal diseases of all types and stages except neural, typhus, some tuberculosis, some leprosy, and influenza leading to death when complicated by bronchial pneumonia. Thus, the need for prevention, particularly sanitation, was evident.

But even education seemed ineffectual in view of the general poverty of the majority. Many of the peasants who crowded the market area could not even afford sandals, which would have reduced hookworm infestation. It is well established in medicine that hookworm in human feces, trampled on the ground where sanitation is lacking, enters the next donor through his bare feet. This dramatic cycle of disease deserves to be highlighted, and the knowledge should be spread to the general population.

This is also one instance in which the role and status of the traditional healers could be employed. They neither object to, nor do they fear the health center. The male healer mentioned above occasionally feels that in some cases his methods are better, e.g. in his herbal shrinking of hemmorhoids which he considers more effective and less troublesome than the surgery recommended by the health officer. Both healers are eager to employ the best practices to care for the people who have confidence in them. This is their ethic as well as their business practice. They are not stubborn and they declare themselves ready to abandon an old practice as soon as they could employ a better one. The female healer sometimes even referred to herself as ignorant (*donkworo*), and to some modern medicines as "beautiful."

Unfortunately, the Health Officer rejects the opportunity of cooperation with these important medical opinion leaders. One reason he gives is that he is very busy with schedules at the clinic. Attendance at the clinic averages 25 patients on ordinary days, and 35 on Mondays. He is most often called away on delivery cases, although he is not trained or equipped to perform Casearian operations. Sometimes he has difficulty in diagnosing cases involving several diseases combined, such as hepatitis combined with relapsing fever. He is often pressured to perform abortions, which he refuses out of fear of legal complications. Friday afternoon is set aside for free treatment of the contagious diseases which the government is most concerned with: tuberculosis, venereal disease, and trachoma. But many female patients and their husbands do not come to this free clinic (to maintain discretion), preferring to attend the regular morning clinic where a fee is charged and where there is less crowding by the very poor. In addition, his time is taken with negotiations with local officials to enlist their cooperation in rabies control by killing suspected dogs; and more of his time is taken up in issuing medical certificates in the numerous litigation cases involving work injuries, accidents,

61

and fights.

But in addition to this well-substantiated shortage of time, the Health Officer in Hosaina and most other places ignores the indigenous healers on the grounds that any attention paid them would enhance the reputation of the traditionalist!

Conclusions and Recommendations

1. The model of the modern Health Center in the small towns of Ethiopia can be evaluated so far only in terms of a pilot project, not in terms of controlling and eradicating disease. He is not yet supported by the necessary economic and educational input that is necessary to break the cycle of reinfection. At the very least every small town receiving a Health Center should also receive a safe water supply, and should manufacture sandals if the people cannot afford to import them.

2. The local elementary school should be the center of the public health effort. The school population is a self-selected elite group in the provincial small town, the reason being that education is not compulsory. Health attitudes of the young can be changed more readily than of the old. The children can be regularly inspected for lice, and they are available to be taught public health methods of human waste disposal, water-boiling and so on. School workshops could start local sandal production. In view of their status, literate students would spread the lessons learned to the poorer youngsters not attending school.

3. Indigenous healers could be the major bridge between the Health Center and the general public, since they already enjoy the personal confidence, availability, and trust associated with the traditional practitioners. This is the most neglected human resource in health care, and it is the least expensive. Their "first aid" practices should be upgraded and their more objectionable practices thereby reduced. In addition, officially recognized and registered indigenous healers would be on the spot to report the outbreak of epidemics, since they would hear of them from peasants in

the remote hinterland. Their employment as opinion leaders to prepare the illiterate and sometimes apprehensive public for vaccination campaigns, e.g., smallpox, which is still a problem in many parts of Ethiopia, is probably essential.

4. Community Nurses should be assigned to mother-child health service only after they themselves have had a child, in view of the general distrust of childless nurses on this subject. Meanwhile, they could work through upgraded female traditional healers.

5. While these conclusions are specifically presented for Ethiopia, many of them can apply also to other rural, undeveloped countries.

6. While the governments of the underdeveloped countries could do more to change the harmful practices of some of the indigenous healers and to replace them with modern medical procedures, little can be gained by denouncing "failure of government to eliminate backwardness." The existence of a predominantly rural population, where no permanent roads exist and illiteracy is very high, presents a syndrome of difficulties. Until these can be resolved, interim improvisations will have to be developed, and this can be done on the local level by these methods of cooperation.

NOTES

Messing, Simon D., "The Highland-Plateau Amhara of Ethiopia." Ph.D. Dissertation, University of Pennsylvania, 1957.

——— "Group Therapy and Social Status in the Zar Cult of Ethiopia," in Opler, M. K. (ed.), *Culture and Mental Health*, Macmillan, New York, 1959.

——— "The Abyssinian Market Town," in *Bohannen and Dalton: Markets in Africa*, Northwestern University Press, 1962.

——— "Application of Health Questionnaire to Pre-urban Communities in a Developing Country." *Human Organization*, Winter, 1965.

——— "Social Problems Related to the Development of Health in Ethiopia." *Social Science & Medicine*, London, 1970, Volume 3, pp. 831-337.

Tseghe, Yohannes, Prince, J.S.: Spruyt, D., "Application of Modern Principles of Public Health Practice to the Solution of Health Problems in Ethiopia." Paper F/37 Principles of Health Service Planning,

F. 1.2. U.N. Conference on Application of Science and Technology for the less Developed Countries. Geneva, E/Conf. 39/Inf. 3, Feb. 4-20, 1963.

World Health Organization Chronicle, *The Smallpox Situation* (Ethiopia). Volume 25, pp. 396-401. September, 1971.

"SCIENTIFIC" PSYCHIATRY AND "COMMUNITY" HEALERS

Enrique Araneta, Jr., M.D.

I. Cultural Psychiatry and the Disease Model

"Cultural Psychiatry," which Dr. Wittkower defines as "that which concerns itself with the mentally ill in relation to their cultural environment within the confines of a given cultural limit,"[1] is not a new field or conceptual approach. It can be traced back to the beginning of this century when Emil Kraeplin in 1904, impressed by the regional differences in psychiatric manifestations in different areas of Europe, set off for Java to study the cultural influences on the frequency and symptomatology of mental disorders in that country.[2] At about that same time, other psychiatrists and social scientists reported and described culture-bound syndromes such as Amok, Latah, the Windigo Psychoses and Artic Hysteria. These studies clearly confirmed that the causation, manifestation and management of "mental" disorders are indeed culturally influenced and defined. However, despite these very impressive and profound observations, interest in the investigation of the cultural assumptions underlying the practice of and research in Psychiatry did not follow. It was not until the second half of this century, when such workers as Ralph Linton, Abraham Kardiner, Margaret Mead, Ruth Benedict, George Devereux and other anthropologists and psychoanalysts called attention to the influence of culture on the modal personality structure and coping styles, that "modern" psychiatry has accorded importance to the study of "cultural factors" in psychiatric illness, and fostered interest in cultural and trans-cultural psychiatry.

Dr. Wittkower and other authorities in the fields of cultural and trans-cultural psychiatry attribute the emergence of this interest to 1) technological advances that brought forth (a) ease in travel, (b) acute awareness of the interdependence of the world in the Nuclear Age and (c) interest in the psychological set and problems in other countries;

2) change in the anthropologists' interest from merely describing socio-cultural institutions to deciphering the whys and hows of their influence on human behavior; and 3) the birth of a new brand of psychiatrists who sought understanding of the dynamics of human behavior beyond the perspective available in the mental hospital grounds or the four walls of their offices. [2]

Although these factors undoubtedly fostered the re-awakening of interest in a cultural approach to the understanding of both normal and abnormal behaviors, they do not explain the long delay in this "re-awakening." I submit that this delay has been due to a large degree to the inability of psychiatrists to look beyond the "disease model" of conceptualizing abnormal behavior. Beset by the political need to reaffirm their identity with the fraternity of "scientific" healers and sensitive to the growing synicism against the arbitrariness of tradition and religion, psychiatrists in the first half of this century very understandably fell into the trend established by the technological age (initiated by the industrial revolution). This scientific trend has led to the assumption, held either overtly or covertly by most psychiatrists, that there exists a universal, scientific psychiatry— a psychiatry that could effectively deal with "mental illnesses" among all peoples, irrespective of their social or cultural backgrounds, just as penicillin deals with pneumonia, anesthesia with pain, or appendectomy with appendicitis.

II. The Medical Metaphor and the Myth of Universal Scientific Psychiatry

A distorted assumption perpetuated by the disease model of conceptualizing psychiatric disorders is embodied in the literal acceptance of the AMA and the APA slogan that "Mental illness is like any other illness." An unfortunate implication of this metaphor is that people's "psyche" or "personality" produce specific responses to particular stresses, as their organs and tissues do. And, since physiology and pathology vary little from one social or cultural group to another, the natural inference is that "personality" functioning and "psychopathology" can be studied and dealt with independently of cultural influences and definitions. It is in this unqualified acceptance of the medical metaphor that the myth of a "universal scientific psychiatry" has been nurtured and continues to "hang on." The pervasiveness of this assumption was well illustrated at a multinational presentation under the Section entitled: "Looking Forward: On the reciprocal interaction of Asian and American Educators," at the APA Annual Meeting in Honolulu, Hawaii, on May 10, 1973. The discussion and exposition presented by the Philippine and Indonesian psychiatrists did not touch on how indigenously-held beliefs and practices influenced their diagnostic and therapeutic approaches, as I had anticipated. Instead, what was focused on were:—how western type psychiatric facilities are being expanded and how western therapeutic approaches are more widely available, in their respective countries. Discussion of rural-dwelling non-westernized patients or indigenous healing practices was omitted. The attitude here reflected, suggests that in actual practice, it is really from the standpoint of a "universal scientific psychiatry" that most disordered behaviors are perceived, evaluated and managed by most psychiatrists. Although this could be assumed to reflect an ethnocentric orientation poetically expressed as "the wine of human nature is everywhere the same, it is only bottled in different labels;" I suspect that professionally conditioned needs and compulsions inherent to medical training contribute significantly to the persistence of this perspective. The need to identify external causes and specific host vulnerability, and the compulsion to "diagnose" disease entities are fixations difficult to overcome, and intrudes against the incorporation of a broader socio-cultural perspective. An unfortunate consequence of this restriction to a "universal, scientific, medical" perspective is that it tends to narrow the focus of therapeutic intervention to the "ill" personality rather than upon the reciprocal interaction between the individual and his life style; and the cultural sanctions and assumptive world within which he seeks his fulfillment. Thus, despite the incorporation of such socially-derived concepts as scapegoating, role-playing, group-process, family-dynamics, social labeling theory, etc. in psychiatric theories and parlance, psychiatric trainees in general, have encountered unwarranted difficulty in expanding their conceptualization and therapeutic versatility because of the paralogism of the medical metaphor. With the introduction and eventual imposition of the institutionalized peer review and hospital guidelines and criteria, one can look forward to further reinforcement of this metaphor and intensified rigidification of conceptual boundaries.

III. The Anthropological Model as "Scientific" Psychiatry

In challenging this widely-held assumption of a "universal scientific psychiatry" that is reflective of the disease model by which most psychiatric disorders are approached, I do not mean to question the reality of associated physiologic (particularly neuro-endocrine) changes occurring with the perception of "psychological stress," or the experience of "emotions." The association of changes in heart rate and blood pressure, and in respiratory, muscular, gastro-intestinal and glandular activities with exposure to psychological stress as described by Cannon and Selye, is beyond question.[3,4,5,6] These measurable changes upon which the polygraph (lie detector) test is based, and on which pharmacalogic and other somatic therapies have proved useful would appear to justify the disease model approach. However, though these changes produce unpleasant sensations, they do not constitute more than mere symptoms of a disordered adjustment, which, in fact, is what we are concerned with when we think of a psychiatric disorder. And I submit that what constitute "psychological stress and disordered adjustment" are culturally defined, and the very way a particular psychological stress is perceived and how the associated physiologic changes are reacted to are culturally determined.[7,8] The reported increasing incidence of sexual impotence among young males since the advent of increased sexual freedom among women in this country illustrates this relationship clearly. This "cultural determinism" is unavoidable since, in dealing with "psychological stresses" and "psychiatric disorders," our concern is really with socially defined "roles" and the "self concept," which are shaped primarily by cultural definition rather than by genetic and biologic (supra-cultural) determination. Thus, Twiggy would likely not feel as pleased with her figure were she in ancient Polynesia.

Therefore, though pharmacologic and other somatic therapies may serve to temporarily alleviate the unpleasant sensations associated with the perception of "psychological" stress, successful adjustment or the attainment of "mental health" does not come about until a mutually-enhancing or -acceptable relationship or interaction is established between the individual and his cultural milieu. The studies of John and Elaine Cummings, in which they showed that the nurses aides' assessment of the social acceptability of a patient proved more reliable than the psychiatrists' evaluation of that patient's intra-psychic integrity in predicting his adjustment of his community, attests to this socio-cultural (anthropological) definition of "mental health."[9]

It follows, therefore, that unlike the usual medical approach to therapy which is directed towards correcting the internal processes within the patient that have gone awry, in Psychiatry our concern is really with the mutually-qualifying interaction between the individual and his milieu. Hence, therapy is more likely to succeed when it is culturally syntonic rather than diagnosis-specific. This has been repeatedly confirmed by reports of transcultural psychiatrists.[10,11,12,13] In my own experience while collaborating with an indigenous (Kali) healer in Guyana; —many cases come to mind that verify this proposition. One such case is that of a young man who rather suddenly developed both conversion symptoms (weak spells with cardiac symptoms) and dissociative episodes in association with a family conflict. The patient's problem was discussed with the Kali healer who, though receptive of the suggested influence of the "family dynamics" on the evolution of the symptoms, nonetheless concluded that the indicated (psychotherapeutic) approach, in accordance with the patient's perception of how his symptoms developed, was to treat the case as one of "possession." Accordingly, after a few days of preparation,

69

including joint family devotions, during which their respective roles in helping the patient overcome his state was clarified, a ritual exorcising the malevolent spirits was undertaken. The patient's symptoms gradually remitted while family communication and relationship improved.

Drs. Wen-Sheng Tseng and John F. McDermott, Jr., in writing on "Psychotherapy: Historical Roots, Universal Elements and Cultural Variations," point out that "different societies will always tend to shape the interpretation of problems according to their own inherent socio-cultural characteristics," and conclude "that the special cultural dimensions of psychotherapy consist of defining cultural norms, reinforcing culturally sanctioned coping mechanisms, and providing "time out" from usual cultural expectations."[10] Dr. Jerome Frank, in writing about common factors in psychotherapy, emphasizes the need for the therapist and patient to start off with a mutually shared belief about the nature of the illness and the treatment process.[14]

These concepts have been used successfully by many western-trained psychiatrists working in unfamiliar cultures, through collaboration with "native" healers.[11,15] In comparing results of the treatment of schizophrenic patients in the villages of Mauritius with comparable patient groups in Great Britain, Nancy Waxler points out that clinical symptoms and social performance after twelve years are significantly better in the former group. She suggests that "beliefs about the nature of the illness constitute the major factor in influencing the prognosis."[16]

From the foregoing discussion, it becomes evident, therefore, that if there is to be a scientific psychiatric approach, it has to be through "cultural" psychiatry. Thus, we find the popularity of mystical and magical rituals among supernaturally oriented cultures, Morita therapy and autogenic training among the highly disciplined and authority oriented Japanese and Germans, work therapy among the work-oriented cultures of the People's Republic of China and the USSR,[13] and analytic psychotherapy among the intellectual elites whose faith is in western rationalism.

Even the idea of transcendence and liberation from cultural deception and bondage alluded to by Dr. Allan

Watts in his book: *Psychotherapy: East and West*, really calls for a conversion to a new, though certainly uncommon belief system. In Dr. Watts' expositions, he traces man's psychological conflicts and miseries to his enslavement to culturally defined roles and expectations. These pressures lead him to pursue "Ego-Enhancing" goals that may be totally irrelevant to ecological harmony or to his biologic economy. The result is conflict, tension, self-deception and confusion. Dr. Watts suggests that by psychoanalysis one transcends cultural definitions by reason, whereas through Eastern process of liberation, the "culture game and self-concept" fades into insignificance before a cosmic consciousness or identity. But, does not this faith and devotion to rationalism or to cosmic consciousness constitute new belief systems or cults? And can one not receptive of the above beliefs benefit from these prescribed procedures? Whatever the case, can one conceive of a cultureless psychiatry?

Drs. H.M. Adler and Van Buren O. Hammot, in writing on the generic factors in all interpersonal therapies in their article entitled: "Crisis, Conversion and Cult Formation,"[17] note that an examination of common psycho-social function, "the placebo effect rests on the universal need of humans for a group, and by symbolic extension,—a system." They conclude that "this common sequence of crisis, conversion, and cult formation. . . .provides a rationale for understanding psycho-analysis, as well as therapeutic communities. In this sense, the psychoanalyst is the priest of a rational system or the charismatic leader of a rational cult."

IV. Community Psychiatry and Indigenous Healers

A major step towards a socio-cultural approach to psychiatry has been afforded by the development of Community Psychiatry. Two major theoretical assumptions gave impetus for advocacy for this approach. First, was that the role obligations and status positions in the community can not be fulfilled and "worded out" in the hospital environment; and, second, that prolonged hospitalization caused the "mentally ill role" to be ingrained. The implication in this new (Community Psychiatry) approach is that modifying behavior to cope effectively with "problems in living" can best be undertaken in the community context; where cultural re-enforcers exert their most meaningful influence on the on-going social processes of role-assigning and role-assuming.

In actual practice, however, Community Psychiatry programs, for the most part, have retained the medical model and has not incorporated to any significant degree the socio-cultural perspective underlying the theoretical basis on which it was conceived. Dr. Paul Roman, Ph.D., discussing the impact of "Psychiatric Sociology" on the ideology and practice of American psychiatry, asserts that "the medical model or disease definition of Psychiatric illness is very evident in much of the ideology and practice of Community Psychiatry." He further states: "The notion that the patient should regard himself as suffering from an emergent 'disease' discontinuous with his normal 'problems in living,' and that he should be treated by an agent with the official medical credentials are a carry-over from traditional hospital Psychiatry, which are evident in Community Psychiatry."

Despite this unfortunate restriction on the input of social scientists on Community Psychiatry programs, a few enterprising psychiatrists, dedicated to the understanding of problems peculiar to their "catchment areas" discovered that the various social and cultural groups within their sphere of responsibility showed variations not only in the frequency, severity and manifestations of "psychiatric impairment," but also in differential response to various treatment modalities. These observations have led to many theoretical speculations and formulations about special behavioral and psychodynamic characteristics of—"the culture of the poor, the Street (drug) culture, the Chicano, Puerto Rican, and other minority cultures." However, little if any constructive and practical therapeutic approaches have been devised, except the utilization of "indigenous workers." The few community psychiatrists that were really determined to work within the cultural context in which their patients lived, suffered and loved embarked upon collaborative working relationship with traditional healers and indigenous workers.[19] This step afforded the effective utilization of appropriate cultural sanctions and re-enforcers, as well as group identification in the "therapeutic process." Much like the collaborative efforts between western-trained psychiatrists and indigenous healers in underdeveloped countries, this approach yielded gratifying therapeutic results and learning experience, in most instances.[20] These successes have resulted in a number of publications, as well as panel discussions in psychiatric and Anthropological Society meetings. Nevertheless, despite the convincing reports of the therapeutic merits of this approach, the number of psychiatric programs that have adopted this collaborative approach to "problems in living" has not significantly increased.

In addition to personality factors, many political, ideological, and ethical issues are involved in this collaborative therapeutic work with traditional healers. This was the focus of the discussion by the panel on "Community Healers and Community Psychiatry" moderated by Joseph Westermeyer, M.D., at the American Psychiatric Association meeting in Detroit, Michigan, in May, 1974.

Whereas, collaboration between western-trained psychiatrists and indigenous healers appear to offer the optimal form of psychiatric care in developing nations, where the economic situation and technological sophistication offer virtually no alternatives;[1,13] the advisability of adopting this measure in the USA has been seriously questioned along the following lines: 1) The difficulty in collaboration would be greater, because the traditional healer who, in this instance, belongs to the minority culture, would be more guarded, expecting the representative of the dominant culture (the powerful psychiatrist) to be more demanding and inflexible. Thus, competition for control of the patient rather than collaboration is more likely. 2) Unlike the situation in the under-developed countries, our traditions and laws exert greater obstacles to the legitimization of the role of the indigenous healer, especially in the attribution of "medical" responsibility. 3) Since there exists no comparable shortage of trained mental health professionals and paraprofessionals with considerable scientific background in social and medical sciences, the use of indigenous healers appears to be no more than a glorified, regressive fad designed to camouflage a type of social exploitation reminiscent of colonialism. 4) Since psychiatrists could not possibly share the unscientific, magical beliefs of the traditional healer, sanctioning the perpetuation of the healing rituals constitutes a prostitution of medicine that is unjustifiable. 5) The perpetuation of unscientific beliefs would foster culture lag that would deter improvement in the standard of living, increased life expectancy and other benefits of increased sophistication in hygienic measures.

These objections can perhaps be reduced to two basic issues. First, does collaboration with indigenous healers provide significantly better therapeutic results in dealing with psychiatric impairment in minority groups and subcultures? And, second, does collaboration with indigenous healers inevitably foster the perpetuation of animistic, magical, supra- and preter-naturally-oriented cultural patterns that have limited capacity to incorporate technological and social progress, resulting in their being delegated to the role of a colonialized minority?

V. Cultural Psychiatry: Colonialism or Community Development

Reports by a number of community psychiatrists, including Ruiz, Bergman, and others show that many patients could never possibly have been brought to treatment were it not for the collaboration of traditional healers. If only for this reason, this collaboration offers definite therapeutic advantages. Additionally, these workers report that patients not responsive to methods of modern psychiatry recover when the therapy is adapted to their culturally bound concept of their illness. Dr. Wittkower, referring to traditional healers in developing countries, says "it cannot be disputed that at least for the treatment of psycho-neuroses, the traditional healer is often effective and, at any rate, the results of western psychotherapy are not staggering."[13] In my own experience in working with a Kali healer in Guyana, I have been impressed by the healer's effectiveness in effecting recovery amongst cases of psycho-physiologic and neurotic disorders, where I had previously failed, utilizing various conventional psychotherapeutic approaches. This underscores the idea previously alluded to, that in psychotherapy what is dealt with is the patient's belief system and conceptual style, which are culturally conditioned, and therefore responsive to culturally defined behavior modifiers, rather than diagnosis specific remedies. Attesting to this is the unanimous assertion by participants of the PAHO/WHO seminar on mental health in Kingston, Jamaica, in 1965, that psychoanalytic psychotherapy was not effective (in indicated disorders) among the non-westernized, native population of the Caribbean countries. It is clear, therefore, that implementing cultural psychiatry with the services of indigenous healers affords superior therapeutic results.

The probability of stunting cultural development by directing therapy towards promoting ethno-cultural adaptation, as opposed to questioning of cultural values and culturally conditioned behavior patterns typical of analytic psychotherapy, would appear theoretically to constitute a disadvantage of cultural psychiatry. That culture change should keep up with technological and socio-economic advances is a hope every community psychiatrist shares. If, indeed, by culturally-oriented psychotherapy we do produce "culture-lag" that will eventually lead to a colonialized cultural group; then, all the therapeutic advantages would be futile, since we would have saved deviant individuals to constitute a deviant group. This would, indeed, be poor community psychiatry. However, does it necessarily follow that by dealing with problems of living in a cultural context in collaboration with indigenous healers, we inevitably stunt culture development? I would question this assumption, since all cultures except those that have been completely isolated have managed to evolve, (even among colonialized nations). It appears that the crucial issue in cultural growth is contact versus isolation, rather than the fact that the members seek their identity and fulfillment within the cultural boundaries, instead of questioning the cultural values. Even the original psycho-analytic group became rigid and stagnant until contact with the dissenting group was re-established. Returning now to the problem of implementing cultural psychiatry thru collaboration with the indigenous healers, it can be deduced that, by collaboration, exchange of ideas and growth is more likely to occur than by avoidance, repudiation and isolation, which is the more commonly assumed stance held by the "scientific purists." In a paper with Dr. Singer, the editor of this volume, "The Learning of Psychodynamics, History, Diagnosis, Management, Therapy, By a Kali Cult Indigenous Healer in Guyana," the expansion of cultural concepts of psychiatric illness and its treatment thru collaboration amongst the Healer, Anthropologist and Psychiatrist is described. By involving the healer in history-taking, diagnostic and management conferences, and by observation and discussion of each other's treatment methods and rationale, the healer became proficient in directing his history taking towards uncovering relevant family- and psycho-dynamic factors, and the covert goals of the patients. The healer even acquired a tape recorder, the better to criticize his interviewing technique, and to more effectively recover and review data. He learned to recognize symptom complexes that suggest physical illness and referred these patients promptly to physicians. Thru collaboration, the healer was able to appreciate the efficacy of E.C.T. and pharmacotherapy, and to recognize and refer those cases that are likely to benefit from these modalities of treatment. Indeed, even the therapeutic regimen for the various conditions that the healer's help was sought, was gradually modified to include opportunities for some family psychotherapy, utilizing family dynamics and group processes that he has learned to apply. The innovations adopted by the healer resulted in expanding the conceptual frame with which he dealt with psychiatric disorders and his relationship with his patients. The patients and their families, in turn, also broadened their conceptualization of emotional and behavioral disturbances. As for the Psychiatrist, he would be writing about electrotherapy instead of this paper had he not had the experience of this collaboration.

The next important question, then, is whether this type

of collaboration can be effected in this country, where the traditional healer belongs to the minority culture. I really see no obstacle to this as long as the practitioner holds a strong conviction about the merits of culturally-oriented psychotherapy. If he has this, he should have no trouble sharing information and responsibility on a peer basis, with mutual respect. Indeed, available papers describing collaborative endeavours, indicate that this is already being achieved.[19,20] This should deter against the tendency to be competitive or to assert dominance. It must always be borne in mind that in psychotherapy, the one most knowledgeable about the patient's culture can best understand his difficulties, needs, beliefs, goals, alternatives and expectations; and, therefore, the one most likely to be of most help.

That collaboration between traditional healers and scientifically trained psychiatrists and physicians can be a force for integrated cultural development and community development is best brought out in the case of the People's Republic of China, where collaborative endeavours have become part of the national policy on health care delivery. By the simultaneous use of herbal medicine, acupuncture and group therapy, the emphasis on the re-establishment of a sense of group, and a "sense of belonging" is achieved.[21,22] Great strides are being reported in public health, especially in the most complete eradication of V.D., and a dramatic reduction in neonatal morbidity and mortality is reported by Dr. Arena of Chapel Hill. The merging of the traditional reverence for children and family life with the liberation of women are feats of cultural accommodation that becomes possible when the traditional and the modern are not allowed to avoid each other.

It is interesting that the revival of traditional medicine in China blossomed after she had risen from colonialization.

Conclusion

This paper attempts to point out that cultural psychiatry is not only scientific, but affords the most effective and rational therapeutic approach in any given setting. In implementing cultural psychiatry by collaboration with traditional Healers, the probability of promoting culture lag which seem apparent in theory is not so in practice. On the contrary, cultural expansion and growth are likely to be enhanced if mutual respect and candor is maintained in the collaborative venture. The type of acculturation that would accrue from such a collaborative relationship would preclude a colonial-type relationship between the more advanced and less advanced cultural groups.

NOTES

[1]"Transcultural Psychiatry in the Caribbean: Past, Present, and Future" by Eric D. Wittkower, M.D., *Amer. J. Psychiat.*, 127:2, August, 1970.

[2]*Recent Developments in Transcultural Psychiatry*, by Eric D. Wittkower, Ciba Symposium on transcultural psychiatry, edited by A.V. De Reudl and Ruth Porter, Little Brown and Co., Boston, 1965.

[3]"Relationship of Physiological Responses to Affect Expression" Oken, D., Grinker, R.R., Heath, H.A. Herz, M., Korchin, S.J., Sabshin, M., and Schwartz, N.B., *Arch. Gen. Psychiat.*, 6:336, 1962.

[4]"Pain, Fear and Anger in Hypertensives and Normotensives, a Psycho-physiologic Study," Schachter, J., *Psychosomatic Medicine*, 19:17, 1957.

[5]"Cognitive, Social and Physiological Determinants of Emotional States," Schachter, S., and Singer, J., *Psychol. Rev.*, 69:379, 1962.

[6]*Psychological Stress and the Coping Process*, Lazarus, R. S., McGraw-Hill, New York, 1966.

[7]"Personality and Physiological Responses to Motion Picture." Roessler, R. and Collins, F., *Psychophysiology*, 6:732, 1970.

[8]"Somatic Response Patterning and Stress: Some Revision of Activation Theory," In *Psychological Stress*, Appley, M. H. and Trumbull, Eds. Appleton-Century-Crofts, New York, 1967.

[9]*Affective Symbolism, Social Norms, and Mental Illness*, John Cummings and Elaine Cummings.

[10]"Psychotherapy, Historical Roots, Universal Elements, and Cultural Variations," Wen-shing, Tseng, and John F. McDermott, Jr., *Amer. J. Psychiat.* 132:4, April, 1975.

[11]"The Therapeutic Process in Cross-Cultural Perspective—A Symposium" Raymund Prince, M.D., pp. 1172, *Amer. J. Psychiatr.* 124:9, Mar., 1968.

[12]"Cross-Cultural Psychotherapy," by William M. Bolman, *Amer. J. Psychiat.*, 124:9, March, 1968

[13]"Cultural Aspects of Psychotherapy," E.D. Wittkower, Hector Warnes, *Amer. J. of Psychotherapy*, (presented at the ninth International Congress of Psychotherapy, Oslo, Norway, June 29, 1973).

[14]"Common Features of Psychotherapy," Frank, J.D., *Aust. N.Z. J. Psychiat.*, 6:30, 1972.

[15]"Patterns of Psychiatric Care in Developing African Countries: The Nigerian Village Program." In *International Trends in Mental Health*, David, H.P., Ed., McGraw-Hill, New York, 1966, pp. 147-53.

[16]"Culture and Mental Illness—A Social Labeling Perspective," by Nancy E. Waxler, Ph.D., *J. of Nervous & Mental Disorders*, Vol. 159:6 Dec. 1974.

[17]"Crisis, Conversion, and Cult Formation: an Examination of a Common Psychological Sequence," by Herbert M. Adler, M.D., and Van Buren O. Hammett, M.D., *Amer. J. Psychiat.*, 130:8. Aug. 1973.

[18]"Psychiatric Sociology and Community Psychiatry," Paul Roman, Ph.D. *Psychiatry*, 1974.

[19]"Puerto Rican Spiritualist View Mental Illness: the Faith Healer as a Paraprofessional," Luchansky, Egri. G., Stokes, *Amer. J. of Psychiat*, 127: 3, Sept, 1970.

[20]"The Case for the Indigenous Therapist," Torrey, E.F., *Archives of Gen. Psychiat;* Vol. 20 pp. 365-373, No. 3.

[21]"Psychiatric Training and Practice in the People's Republic of China?" by Phillip D. Walls, Lichun Han Walls, & Donald G. Langsley, *Amer. J. Psychiat.* 132:2, Feb. 1975.

[22]"Psychiatry in Shanghai, China: Observations in—1973," by David Ratnavale, M.D., *Amer. J. Psychiat.*, 130:10, October, 1973.

THE ANCIENT ART OF FOLK HEALING: AFRICAN INFLUENCE IN A NEW YORK CITY COMMUNITY MENTAL HEALTH CENTER

Pedro Ruiz, M.D. and John Langrod, M.A.

As Western man continues to unravel the secrets of nature and to transform his discoveries into technology it would appear that the schism between pure and applied science has narrowed; abstract theory has been beaten into the plowshares of practical tools for everyday comfort; logically, mankind in the "developed" countries should have arrived at a universal *mens sana in corpore sano*. At the very least he should be better off. But is he? And if so, by whose criteria?

Even allowing for the unequitable distribution of the world's good things, a visitor from another planet might marvel at the number of unhappy, confused, disoriented and otherwise disabled humans roaming the cities in search of something—identity, meanings—some aspects of their humanity which got lost in the forced march of science and technology. Those of us in the field of mental health are confronted daily with the consequences to individuals of a world whose agenda for the good life is articulated in terms of gross national product rather than in measurements of human happiness or well-being.

This paper will attempt to describe the experience of a community mental health center in the southeast Bronx section of New York City, where modern medical science has come face-to-face with the practice of *espiritismo*, *santeria*, and *brujeria* among the predominantly Spanish-speaking population. Most members of the core mental health professions (psychiatrists, psychologists, nurses and social workers) are trained in the perspectives of the Anglo-European culture and in the medical model, which strives to diagnose and treat symptoms by what they consider to be value-free criteria. But this presupposes a common ground of understanding in a given cultural context.

Even in such a context, science has not been able to define except in the extreme, "mental health" and "mental illness." What we do know is that, as Kiev[1] points out, from birth onward, an individual's biological functions are molded to culturally prescribed limits, and patterned after accepted models and shared attitudes within his cultural milieu. We also know that a sudden move into another cultural environment can cause emotional disturbance and, on a continuum of reaction, approach serious psychological trauma.

In the dilapidated area of the southeast Bronx, the Lincoln Community Mental Health Center serves a population of close to 200,000 people, all of them poor and most of them coming from Hispanic Caribbean countries which still hold to manners, mores and belief systems associated with a pre-industrial world. In that world, a man is usually sustained by an inner spiritual life as important to him as his material existence. This sense of awe toward the spiritual values in life is in marked contrast to post-industrial man's concentration on material goods, scientific "proofs," and only a nod for organized religion. In fact, as Nelson and Torrey[2] have eloquently remarked, functions traditionally recognized as being in the domain of religion have been increasingly assumed by mental health practitioners. But for the Spanish-speaking population of the south Bronx, religious and healing functions are still fused in folk healers; at the same time, people of Hispanic origin for the most part affiliated with the Roman Catholic Church, are also clients of modern health care facilities. How can such disparate bodies of belief and practice be carried all at once?

As a responsible public agency charged with prevention of mental illness as well as its treatment for a whole catchment area, the administration of Lincoln Community Mental Health Center needed to study the different sub-cultures represented there and in particular to examine the methodologies of the folk healers among them. However, before we describe what we found in the various cultural practices, it will be useful for the reader to know how the mental health center functions.

The Lincoln Community Mental Health Center Background

The Community Mental Health Centers Act passed by

the U.S. Congress in 1963 promised a "bold new approach" to mental health services. Importantly, it provided for psychiatric services to be made available to communities— particularly to people in low-income communities—who heretofore had been denied access to professional attention. Based on this philosophy, the Lincoln Community Mental Health Center organized its structure to provide innovative treatment approaches such as the use of teams composed of the core mental health professionals plus a new category of worker—the non-professional—drawn from the community itself, whose knowledge and experience of the area was to serve as a bridge between local residents' needs and traditional practice. An interdisciplinary "New Careers" program was launched to train these workers who were to function under the supervision of professional personnel.

For the first time, maintenance of the mental health of a whole community, rather than the treatment of mental illness of a defined patient, was stated as a goal. This implied a need to understand family, community and cultural norms as well as biological and psychic structures of individuals; and the Center was to encourage community participation in planning and setting priorities for programs.

To make these goals more effective the Lincoln Mental Health Center established satellite centers in local neighbor-hoods manned by teams of mental health workers. Each team was composed of one social worker, one psychologist and four or five nonprofessionals; the shortage of psy-chiatrists resulted in a ratio of only two psychiatrists for an average group of 25,000 of the population. Moreover, psychiatrists were usually engaged in consultation or in training, leaving very little time for actual treatment of patients. Furthermore, medically-trained psychiatrists most often came from a different socio-economic class and a different culture. Their lack of information about Hispanic cultural norms meant that, when they *did* see patients, the diagnoses were almost invariably some form of schizo-phrenia; treatment some form of psychotropic drug. More and more the responsibility for actually helping the people of the southeast Bronx fell on the shoulders of nonprofess-ionals who were part of the community and understood the problems of the new arrivals.

For Puerto Ricans in New York who constitute the majority of the Lincoln Community Mental Health Center clientele, the expectations of a better life which brought them here have given way to the realities of prejudice, language barriers and poverty in a dilapidated area of an indifferent city. The disillusion and culture shock experienced by migrants under such circumstances can cause almost un-bearable stress, hardly conducive to respect and admiration for the new place or its institutions. In such a perceived hostile environment, the new arrival finds reassurance and relief from anxiety by closing ranks with his fellow migrants and holding fast to familiar ways. More than ever he needs to call on his inner spiritual resources to sustain him, and when these fail, to seek the help of Hispanic folk healers.

At the same time, people feel the need for health services available through government-sponsored centers. The result was that, as we discovered, the same patients who were coming into the mental health center in the day time were seeking help from folk healers in the evening. The evidence was all around us: not only did patients repeatedly report that they heard "voices"; but an "evil spirit" was influencing them. On almost every street in certain areas of this district there were "botanicas" which sold herbs and items foreign to the pharmacopeia of an ordinary drug store. On one block within 100 feet of each other, one can ob-serve a mental health center, a storefront church, and a privately organized medical group. Obviously, treatment processes were overlapping. We had to explore the parallel systems if we were to serve our patients realistically. With the help of some of our own nonprofessional employees, we set out to learn about folk healing practices. What we found revealed that we needed to know more about the various subcultures represented in the area; more than that, folk healing practices which were common to certain Caribbean or South American countries were undergoing subtle but significant changes as they came in contact with a revitalized African influence.

Folk-healing Practices in the South Bronx

The majority of the Spanish-speaking population in this area are Puerto Rican in origin, and the predominant folk healing practice there is called *espiritismo.*

Briefly stated, *espiritismo* assumes an invisible world of spirits of people who are either recently dead or dead for many years, who are in the process of delivering themselves from various levels of purgatory into Divine acceptance. For a multitude of reasons having to do with their former lives, the spirits attach themselves to the living and influence them for good or evil. In order to commune with these super-natural forces—to encourage help from the "good" spirits, and ward off trouble from the "evil" spirits—certain members of the community have developed *facultades*—ways of getting directly in touch with the spirit world. These are mediums, or *espiritistas.* They usually developed their *facultades* by undergoing a series of experiences called *pruebas* or tests of faith, after which they may have had a revelation; finally they have emerged with the ability to divine problems of others and to influence different spirits to help them. People who develop spiritual faculties can become mediums, pro-viding they receive a "call" and they believe strongly enough. This usually takes a long time and a great deal of concentrated effort, along with help from established mediums. The practice is regarded by these mediums as a combination of religion and science brought together for the purposes of healing.

Folk healers practice in *Centros,* which are usually store-fronts or rented halls where regular seances are held. Almost all of these are licensed as churches, with regular membership and a president, who is a medium. A smaller *Centro* may be located in the home of the *espiritista.* As many as fifty or more people, or as few as five or six may be gathered for the seance, which is opened with prayers and readings. Ritual gestures are performed, sometimes incense is lighted to encourage the arrival of the spirits. When a client with a problem comes to a meeting at the *Centro* (usually at the urging of and accompanied by relatives or friends) he or she is helped to present the problem by answering questions posed by assembled mediums who may also enter a trance-like state in which they see visions, or *evidencias* concerning the patient's problem. Very often the symptoms described are familiar and persistent physical discomforts. Sometimes the problem is as concrete as an argument with a landlord or contretemps with municipal bureaucracy. No problem is too small to merit attention; the mediums know from experience that certain minor symptoms or events are accompanied by great anxiety. Aided by spirit guides, the mediums probe to discover whether the problem stems from "material" or "spiritual" causes. If the cause is deemed "material" the client is referred to a doctor. Very often, however, the sufferer has already been to a doctor who has been able to find nothing wrong with him. In this case, whatever the symptoms, the problem is considered to be a "spiritual" one, and the spirits will have to be "worked" to cure it. Sometimes the problem is found to be both material and spiritual and both systems of help are advised. Most folk healers have great respect for medical science. However, they believe that since some disorders may be caused by spirits, they should be treated by people who are experienced in dealing with the spirit world. It should be mentioned here that *espiritismo* as practiced in the Hispanic culture differs from English-American spiritualism, which is interested in psychic phenomena, and the development of telepathic faculties. *Espiritismo* is oriented towards the application of spiritual powers to the practical task of healing the afflicted.

We would like to present a detailed account of one seance which we videotaped at a *Centro* in the Bronx. From the outside it looked like an ordinary storefront; on the altar, there are candles and statues of Catholic saints, as well as fruit, water, hanging herbs and corn. Beside the altar is a record player for drum music; a large symbolic religious statue resembling an American Indian stands at the side. On the mediums' table, which is covered with a white cloth, there is a book of prayer, several different colored necklaces (each one representing a different saint); a vase of flowers, vials of perfume and the very important, glass of water. Also hanging on the wall to the side is a horseshoe, with the open end down. One can only speculate what the horseshoe represents; in some rural parts of the United States a horseshoe hung over a door, *open end up*, stands for good luck.

There are several full mediums dressed in white with red scarves tied at the neck, around the table; mediums-in-training sit nearby along the wall. Each of the mediums wears different colored necklaces, which represent the saints the medium has adopted as his or her special guardians. A recording of African drum playing opens the service. The beat is distinctly African, and the purpose is to induce the arrival of spirits at the seance. In Cuba, Puerto Rico, Haiti and other Caribbean countries, live drums are still used; it is a special skill and difficult to learn, therefore good drummers are highly valued, though they are not paid. This is followed by collective praying, with all standing. These are ritual prayers to please the gods and *protecciones*. Following the collective praying a basket is passed for contributions which in this case are used only for maintenance of the church. After this there are individual prayers, also to induce the spirits. Then, because induction of spirits may cause the arrival of bad spirits, a "cleansing" ceremony takes place. Gestures are used to ward off these spirits, also fire and the spreading of perfumed water. With the hands, the medium symbolically grasps the bad spirit and places it in the glass of water on the table. Incense is used both to improve spiritual vision and to induce the favored spirits to arrive. Singing and chanting takes place; in this case in Spanish. During these ceremonial activities, the trainee mediums take part and observe. Occasionally the head medium will call one of the trainees to the table for some part of the service. While performing, he will be observed, and will get a critique of his performance. After the seance is over, trainees can question the mediums and learn what happened; in this way mediums provide ongoing supervision of their trainees.

The second part of the seance consists of consultations. Anyone in the audience who has a problem is invited to the table for help in solving it. The head medium assigns one of the assisting mediums to each case, with assignments rotating around the table. On this occasion, the first client complained that he could not sleep. The medium listens, then goes into a trance, discovers that the angry spirit of a relative is causing the trouble—partly because the person doesn't remember him. The client is advised to satisfy this spirit by becoming more pious; he is to create an altar in his home, offer water, fruit and prayers.

The next consultee complains of depression. Another medium divines that a dead relative misses him and wants him to die and join him. In this case the spirit resists attempts to make him leave. Another medium takes over; the problem is severe. Finally the medium, responding to the client's suicidal feelings, points to his wife and children and their need for him. Thus guilt is brought into the proceedings; the man must not only fight off this spirit, he must think of those who depend on him for material sustenance as head of the household.

A third volunteer is a young single woman who complains of nightmares. The working medium explains that a spirit is trying to get close to her, but doesn't know how because she is not ready. A fourth client is a woman with painful joints. She had been treated repeatedly by doctors at the Lincoln Hospital, and has had medication for the pain, but it doesn't help. This is her first visit to a *Centro;* she is desperate. The medium decides that the problem is indeed "material" but also that there are some spiritual influences at work, and advises the patient to continue with medication and also prescribes special baths for the patient to take at home. Another client, very depressed, cannot be helped by the assembled mediums. She will have to come back for a special individual consultation with the head medium.

At the end of the session there is a cleansing dance, accompanied by singing and the drums. Everyone takes part, including the observing public and young children. One female child only seven years old appears to enter a deep trance with violent continuous movements of hands and feet and head which might seem alarming (almost like an epileptic fit) to an outsider. In this group it indicates that she is developing spiritual powers very early. We got permission from the president of the church and the mother to examine the girl at home, and found her free of psychopathological signs.

In this particular *Centro*, the head medium is a man who was studying to be a Roman Catholic priest when, in his last year of study, he had a revelation. He lived with his aunt, a very pious Catholic lady. One day a person came to the door asking for food. He was obviously starving. The aunt refused to give him food. The young student priest was shaken; he questioned the value of a religion whose pious adherents would refuse a starving man food. He searched for a better way, and found that *espiritismo* with its empathic approach to human dilemmas, came closer to the real meaning of a religious life.

The seance described above, held regularly in a *Centro*, is open to anyone who cares to come in. Another form of spiritualist practice which we investigated in our neighborhood departs from *espiritismo* practice in some important ways. The syncretic cult of *santeria*, known to be the most prevalent in Cuba, is considered to have even more African influence than *espiritismo*.

To begin with, the santeria session which we observed was closed to the public. The senior medium, in this case a Cuban lawyer and sociologist, is known as the *Babalao*, similar to the head medium or president of the spiritualist *Centro*. The belief system is rooted in the concept of rebirth in the *Lucumi* religion; the use of African drums and animal sacrifice is part of secret rituals to induce help from African gods. In this case, statues of the gods on the altar are dressed like the Catholic saints; but they are black and have names such as *Obatala*, *Oshun*, *Yemaya* and *Shango*. The ceremony we witnessed was for the purpose of helping a female patient who had a three-year history of stomach problems; X-rays and treatment at Lincoln Hospital as well as from several private practitioners had not helped her. She had been advised by a friend to consult the *Babalao*, and he had divined a spiritual cause for her difficulty. The ceremony, which took some days to prepare was conducted in the back of a store-front *botanica*. It was set for a Sunday morning at 11:00 A.M. and lasted until 6:30 P.M. The *Babalao* has several assistants, and there are trainees present, but trainees are allowed to see only part of the ceremony.

Preparations include a special bath, made up of water,

grated coconut meat mixed with herbs; a necklace especially prepared for the patient to wear for life; a bowl of a farina mixed with the meat of three chickens of different colored feathers. The chickens have been killed and their blood collected as part of the ceremony. At the back of the altar are preparations of food and drink for a party, if the therapeutic ritual results in a successful outcome.

The patient takes off her clothes and the ritual of the bath is performed. This is accompanied by drums and praying. She drinks some of the blood of the sacrificed animals and eats some of the farina. Symbolically the blood will push out the offending elements causing the stomach problems while the farina will protect the stomach wall from further ailments.

To make a stronger case for her recovery, everyone present participates in each step of the ceremony including the drinking of some of the animals' blood. This is followed by a toast to the gods in whiskey and wine, the smoking of cigars; in the cult of *santeria*, the members do what they believe the gods would want to do if they were on earth, in order that, through identification, the gods will be more powerfully influenced to aid a client.

When the prayers and ceremony are finished, the *Babalao* throws four broken coconut shells; the manner in which they fall will decide whether the ceremony was conducted properly. If the sign is one of recovery, some members of the sect which meets in this *botanica* will be called to come for a party. The chickens and the farina will be cooked and eaten; fruit is passed; drinks are served; a full celebration takes place. Each action during the celebration has a special meaning. This day-long ritual is offered at no cost to the patient. However, she must pay for the fruit, chickens, and liquor which will be needed for the ceremony.

It is generally acknowledged that the *santeria* cult, with its African emphasis, is spreading among the Puerto Rican *espiritistas* in practice in the area. From an outsiders' standpoint, the difference between the two spiritualist cults would seem to be that *espiritismo* is mainly concerned with healing, or solving problems, by "working through" the spirits. *Santeria*, appears to be less concerned with symptoms and more on the other hand, with emphasis on re-birth and an identity with African gods—all of this as a process of growth and personal development.

Those of us with scientific training will inevitably try to find codified rules in the rituals, and seek to identify treatment modalities with what we practice in the mental health profession. But it is important to remember that all of these folk healing cults are flexible; espiritualistic leaders may incorporate at will new artifacts or religious items or ideas into their ceremonies. The point is that whatever appears to work is acceptable, there is none of the rigidity one associates with organized religion or with organized science, for that matter. The eclectic nature of the folk healer systems make it possible for them to accept, however, the possibility that professional mental health workers, such as psychiatrists, psychologists and social workers, also may have a useful role in healing the afflicted. A discussion with a practicing *espiritista*, who is also a nonprofessional health worker at the Lincoln Community Mental Health Center, reveals some of the philosophical underpinnings which make it possible to accept both systems, and more.

From the Espiritista Point of View

Aida H. . .is an American-born Puerto Rican in her forties with a pleasant, open, animated manner and an attractive face and figure. She of course was aware of spiritualists in her youth but in fact did not go to a *Centro* or have any contact with them until her late thirties. At that time because the chemicals were giving her a bad reaction, she had to give up her profession as a hairdresser. She had a dream about an old man who was dead, but got up and walked. It was of course the biblical Lazarus. He seemed to be trying to tell her something; the dream had such force that she wanted to consult a spiritualist at once, but her husband forbade it. She had the dream several times more, and finally defied her husband and set up an altar in her home. She began to meet with three friends on a regular basis to meditate and read prayers, and together they would go to

90

church. Gradually, Aida developed her spiritual powers, and was able to help others.

When the Lincoln Community Mental Health Center opened and was looking for community people whom they could train as nonprofessionals, Aida was found qualified and hired. From the vantage point inside the Center, she was able to see the methods used by psychiatrists, and she could see where they failed to help. She could also recognize the kind of psychiatric help which was beneficial, and saw no reason why the two systems could not be used simultaneously.

According to Aida, spiritual healing comes down to a matter of faith. There is such a thing as magic; it cannot be explained. "Society," says Aida, "can kill you. Some can cope more than others, a good medium can be very helpful. They cannot always cure the problem, but they can fortify one to the point where he can deal with himself; he can function." In addition to faith a good medium must have humility and generosity of spirit. Aida is aware that there are charlatans in operation in the area, too. She tells of the case of Maria S. . ., whose son was a drug addict with a record of mugging and stealing to pay for his habit. She brought him to the Center (after getting no help from other agencies); where they convinced him that he should go to Lexington, Kentucky to be cured. Maria put him on the bus, but after four or five days he left and came home. Maria became a prostitute in order to support his habit and keep him out of trouble. Aida made a home visit to Maria, who told her she had dreams, heard people talking; she felt she was undergoing a *prueba*. Aida accompanied Maria to a *Centro*, where the room was darkened; a black coffin stood in the middle of the room; people, in turn would get into the coffin and the medium (male) would pass a red handkerchief a few times around the coffin and be ready for the next one. Aida did not react as a medium; she did not become involved; she told Maria that this was not a true *espiritismo*; he was hypnotizing people in the coffin but he was not in touch with the spirits, and what's more, he charged for the service and this exposed him as a charlatan, because real spiritualists are never commercial. Aida took Maria to a home type seance held by an elderly Puerto Rican woman. There Maria learned to pray, found faith, set up an altar in her home, all in hopes of getting her son off drugs. It took a long time, but she kept at it, and says Aida, today her son is stabilized on methadone, is married and has two children. Maria met some Haitians at the *Centro* and later went to Haiti to make her *ocha*. The *ocha* is a ceremony in *santeria* practice which helps you to get in touch with your guardian angel. Everyone has a guardian; your own must be discovered. The day this happens is celebrated on its anniversary every year. Maria is now a practicing *espiritista*, remarried to a good man, and functioning very well. Her diagnosis by the doctor was schizophrenia.

In another case, Rosa was brought to the emergency room of the Lincoln Hospital bleeding from a beating her husband had given her. She had been found walking the streets barefooted in her nightgown. The doctor diagnosed her as unstable, insecure, suffering from social and marital problems. She (the doctor) prescribed the tranquilizer Valium, but realized the woman needed help which medicine could not provide, and referred her to Aida, who helped with housing, welfare, and other practical needs that she had. At the same time, she helped her spiritually with prayers and introduced her to her own guiding spirit—Lazarus—to whom Rosa became devoted. This case, too, had a good outcome, and Rosa is now functioning well.

According to Aida, some doctors are still in the psychosis bag, and feel you can only dominate the mind with medication. She feels that if you have nothing better to give the patient than drugs, you're not doing anything. With drugs alone, a person may function to a certain level. But the side effects of the drugs might render the patient in a worse condition than the former psychosis. Further drug side effects may even hamper full rehabilitation. On the other hand, some cases, according to Aida, are so deteriorated that you can't use spiritualism, and the *espiritista* must know the cut-off point, when the only answer is hospitalization.

Aida is not dismayed by the incursion of *santeria* practices in so many of the *Centros*. The African gods are powerful because they relate to natural forces such as earth, fire and water. The sacrificing of animals occurred in the Scriptures, as did the unexplained miracles like Lazarus returning from the dead. A real *santero* will practice *santeria* only, and its origins are African. *Espiritistas* (Aida believes 90% of them), who rely on meditation and believe in reincarnation, also feel that the "seven great African powers" are important spiritual factors. With all due respect to medical research, Aida is strong in her conviction that no amount of research can completely explain the mysteries of the human condition in terms which satisfy the rational mind. As Aida puts it, "We have a spiritual side to our nature which can be tapped for help, but only if you have faith."

The Dilemma of Mental Health Professionals

The methodologies in treatment used by modern psychiatry have broadened to include group process, family and milieu therapy, psychodrama and other methods comparable to the group approach of the *Centros*. But it should be remembered that most institutions training psychiatrists still base their didactic and practicum training on the classic model, which calls for a good deal of introspection and verbal ability on the part of the patient. Such training is scientifically oriented and ethnocentric, in that it holds to Anglo-European cultural values and belief systems. Therefore it must categorically deny the existence of supernatural influences. Yet a belief in such influences is imbedded in Hispanic culture; and it is in the cultural differences that the problem ultimately rests. Some investigators of folk healing practices have tried to link such methods with those used in psychiatry. Lubchansky et al.[3] for example, in observing an *espiritista* seance in the Bronx was able to translate the process of diagnosis and treatment into psychiatric terms involving the super-ego, the ego and the id. Kiev[4] compared the relative merits of the Mexican folk healing system (*curanderismo*) and dynamic psychotherapy and found both systems beneficial under certain circumstances, concluding that the differences were due not to scientific factors but to cultural ones. The *espiritista* Aida, consulted for this study, saw no dichotomy in her dual role as a mental health worker supervised by psychiatrists and as an *espiritista*. For her, the patients' problems are either "material"—needing medical attention, or "spiritual"—needing help from spiritualists; or possibly, problems may have elements of both, needing help from both types of practitioners. In either case, practitioners, to have a successful outcome, should be aware of the cultural context of the patient. In the Lincoln Community Mental Health Center we have come to realize that for the majority of our Spanish-speaking population, folk healers are an important part of their lives and social network. While we cannot arrive at the synthesis of ideologies, we can and do work with folk healers in trying to help our patients.

It is interesting to note, however, that social pressures to assimilate are strong in this Anglo-dominated society, yet *espiritismo* appears to be reaching out towards Africa for its symbols and rituals, rather than to the accepted shibboleths or status symbols which characterize the American belief system. The examination of this phenomenon would make an interesting sociological research project; here we can only speculate that the African gods have come to represent great strength in the spirit world, and the condition of the most newly-arrived Hispanics in New York is so desperately powerless that even the *protecciones* of *espiritismo* need reinforcement. As Aida puts it, "When you have very big problems, you need very heavy gods, so you call on the seven great African powers."

Conclusion

Pure science has never had to consider cultural norms or even humanistic values in its pursuit of knowledge. Current research in biochemistry and genetics may provide evidence of brain function and heredity as agents in emotional illness quite apart from psychodynamic factors. But as soon as we move away from what can be discovered by technology about an individual's physical condition, we are in the realm of theory and applied techniques, which is why we have so many divergent schools of psychiatric practice, from chemotherapy to primal screams. What we may be seeing here in the Bronx is a closing of the circle. From one-to-one therapy in the Viennese mode, to community psychiatry and group process; to the introduction of nonprofessionals in the mental health field (by default, as not enough professionals were available); to simultaneous proliferation of *espiritismo* in the same community being served by accredited mental health centers; to the movement of *espiritismo* towards ancient African practices.

What it comes down to is that medically-trained psychiatrists must learn more about the culturally-sanctioned and accepted values men live by, if they are to promote a mentally healthy society. Science has not probed all the corners of the human psyche, nor learned to distinguish how different cultures view the same symptoms; much is still a mystery. Torrey[5] has pointed out that the techniques used by Western therapists in the field of psychiatry are no more nor less "scientific" or "magical" than those used by witch-doctors, and we may have a lot to learn from them. At the same time, modern medicine has certain reliable tools in its armamentarium which can be usefully applied by folk healers, if those tools are put in their hands. In the southeast Bronx, folk healers who also serve in the mental health centers have successfully synthesized both systems. It is perhaps time for the elitist professionals to climb down from their theoretical pedestals and confront the reality of alternative lifestyles and patterns of healing which have worked over the centuries.

NOTES

[1]Kiev, A.: *Curanderismo*, New York, The Free Press, 1968, p. 175.

[2]Nelson, S. H.; Torrey, E. F.: "The Religious Functions of Psychiatry," *American Journal of Orthospsychiatry*, 43 (3): 362-367, 1973.

[3]Lubchansky, I.; Egri, G.; Stokes, J.: "Puerto Rican Spiritualists View Mental Illness: The Faith Healer as a Paraprofessional," *American Journal of Psychiatry*, 125: 312-321, 1970.

[4]Kiev, *op. cit.* p. 186.

[5]Torrey, E. F.: "What Western Psychotherapists Can Learn From Witch Doctors," *American Journal of Orthopsychiatry*, 42 (1): 69-76, 1972.

COLLABORATION WITH TRADITIONAL HEALERS: NEW COLONIALISM *AND* NEW SCIENCE

Joseph Westermeyer, M.D.

I. Introduction

The Topic. Our theme in this essay does not concern just traditional healing *per se.* Rather it addresses purposeful utilization of traditional healing by government agencies, or conscious collaboration with traditional healers by physicians and other "modern"* health care workers. Thus we are discussing a dynamic relationship that involves not just traditional healers themselves, but also government officials with a responsibility for the public's health, professional health care workers and—most importantly—patients and the population at large.

The topic also infers the existence of two separate groups besides traditional healers. One of these is a group of people who want the services of traditional healers. The other group, composed of public health officials and "modern" health care workers (to be abbreviated as HCW) who *presumably*—but so far, not very demonstrably—have it in their power to utilize or collaborate with traditional healers. The former might be an educated elite, a dominating ethnic majority, or a wealthy "industrialized"** society, or

---

*"Modern" is placed in quotes because much of what is subsumed under "modern" or "scientific" medicine is actually quite traditional and empirical. Everyday principles of medical practice and fairly sophisticated observations in physical diagnosis stem back to the Greek, Roman, or Arabian Empires. Numerous commonly used drugs were employed by folk herbalists on all continents long before they were adapted by literate physicians. Some of the earliest surgical innovations originated from barber-surgeons. Even the relationship between healers and patients has changed little from culture to culture, or century to century—whether considered from a legal, ethical, transactional, or methodological perspective.

**The judgemental aspects of these terms perturb me. How is a rural farming society with no unemployment less "industrialized" than an urban factory society with many unemployed people? "Industrialized" for whom, and why, and how? Or is a society that trades illiteracy for vandalism, or malaria for obesity, somehow more "developed"?

an international consortium. The latter might be an ethnic minority, a peasant or tribal population, or members of a "developing"** society.

And finally, the theme infers that there is a judgement to be made. Either such utilization or collaboration should be considered as a form of colonialism, with all the negative connotations of that term. Or it should be considered as science, with the positive—or at least neutral—values that accompany this word. Of course, the built-in recommendation of the theme is that one ought to abandon collaboration with traditional healers because that is a neo-colonialist strategy, or argue for such collaboration because it is scientific. While either alternative might well be desirable, these two alternatives might not exhaust the available alternatives. Thus, we should see whether we can be less swayed by connotation and whether other alternatives or issues might be operative.

Definition of Terms. The traditional healer, for purposes of this paper, will include shaman, spirit or witch doctor, and herbal doctor. Their training ordinarily consists of apprenticeship to an older healer. The conceptual basis for their practice is the theological-philosophical world view of their cultural peers. Ordinarily their powers to heal stem from preternatural powers possessed by or at the disposition of the healer. The knowledge and origins of powers possessed by the healer are ordinarily kept secret. By and large the healer can function only within his/her own ethnic group, since the shared "world view" of both healer and patient are usually integral to the traditional healing process.

Modern health care workers include physicians, dentists, nurses, and other similarly trained practitioners. Their training takes place in colleges or universities under the direction of a group of faculty members. The Scientific Method comprises the basis of their training, supplemented by clinical traditions whose use has usually not been countermanded by (or has been supported by) scientific study. Their information and procedures are shared with colleagues, and tend to be eclectic rather than irrevocably tied to traditional prescriptions. Their powers to heal are based on demonstrated knowledge and skills, certain minimum experience, licensure by the state, and certification by peer professionals.

For a wide range of health problems, the modern HCW often functions well among ethnic groups different from his own (i.e. efficacy does not inevitably depend upon a shared world view between healer and healed).

New colonialism (or neo-colonialism) is always used in the context of more developed or industrialized or wealthy nations doing something to developing or rural or poor nations. Thus, the Japanese contrive to have others depend on them for motorcycles, radios, and watches. Communist nations seek to export their economic theory and political structure "for the good of the proletariat." Western democracies want others to employ democratic social institutions, open their doors to trade, and increase their per capita income. In a very definite sense, these are the same sorts of things that the modern HCW or public health official seeks to do to groups who are using traditional healers. That is, they seek to help these latter peoples attain decreased mortality, increased longevity, decreased morbidity, increased productivity —i.e. "the good life" as the modern HCW conceives it. Thus, any kind of activity by a modern HCW in a traditional society is a form of neo-colonialism, whether or not collaboration occurs with traditional healers. Perhaps, however, there are degrees and kinds of neo-colonialism, some being "better" and some "worse." Of course this raises political and ethical issues (about which more further on).

"New Science" is a contradiction in terms. Science is never new in the sense that its fundamental principles do not change over time. Or it is always new in the sense that it inevitably must address new problems, create new hypotheses, develop new methods. For purposes of this paper, though, it may be well to think of the use of traditional healers for scientifically valid reasons rather than for sentimental or revisionist reasons.

Framing the Appropriate Questions

Health activities inevitably involve political, ethical, and individual issues (Haggerty, 1972; Westermeyer, 1972). In undertaking such activities across social class or ethnic

98

boundaries, the modern HCW must ask, and answer certain
critical questions:

> Why is this agency or group funding me to work
> among the people receiving health care? political
> reasons? missionary zeal? treaty obligations?

> Why am I working among or trying to change other
> than my own people? for money? for adventure?
> for greater prestige in my own reference group? as
> an escape?

> What does the recipient group want me to do for
> them? Why are they willing to receive my assistance?
> to be polite? because other nations have similar
> services? as part of an integrated plan to improve
> their citizens' well being?

These questions must be faced honestly and directly.
Failure to do so can adversely affect both the "helper" (by
disappointing one's expectations) and the "helpee" (by
producing more problems than are alleviated).

Probably the first of these three sets of questions is
answered by most HCW leaving their own culture or social
class to work among a group different from themselves. The
second may be answered in some cases, but—from my own
discussions with many HCW active in such work—is probably
no better understood than are the motivations of HCW in
general as they choose their vacation and go about their work.
The third may never be made explicit, or even ever be discovered by the HCW.

In my first public health venture to Laos in 1965, I knew
from the start who was paying me (the U.S. Agency for
International Development) and why (ostensibly humani-
tarian, but largely political reasons). I had carefully thought
out—even written down—my reasons for seeking such an
experience: cross cultural experience in the health field for
academic reasons, quasi-messianic motivations as a professional "helper" or "do-gooder," and patriotic pro-Ameri-
canism 1965 style (in that order of priority). However, the
third set of questions did not become apparent to me for
about a year. And until it could be answered, my comfort
and effectiveness in my role were both impaired.

In my second cross cultural public health activity I was

careful to attend to all three sets of questions. The second time around I learned much faster. It became evident in about one month that the funding agency (a federal bureaucracy) actually had no interest in the desires of the recipient group (plains American Indians), but only in mollifying a political figure (a U.S. senator) and in aggrandizing the agency (Westermeyer and Hausman, 1974).

In several public health activities since then, I find myself to be increasingly astute in avoiding all involvement in undertakings where the goals of the recipient group have been ignored, or not sought, and simply absent or assigned no priority by the recipient group.

History provides us with two common dilemmas which have resulted from ignoring these important questions. In the first case, a physician has left his own industrialized country to emigrate into a tribal or peasant society. More specifically, white Western men have gone to black and brown peoples in Africa and Asia: Seagraves to Burma, Schweitzer to Africa, Dooley to southeast Asia. In retrospect none of these physicians had a lasting impression on the indigenous health care system. Once the charismatic leader died, his organization atrophied. The health of the recipient population was not improved by the effort—and neither was it much hindered. In toto, the effect was not improved health for the recipient population, but rather an adventure for the donor.

The second case is perhaps less known, less dramatic, but certainly more destructive to the recipient population. No charismatic leaders are associated with such efforts—indeed, none of the individuals involved is widely known. Unlike the primary physicians in the former group, they were public health officers, sanitarians, administrators, and engineers. They drained swamps, eliminated malaria, provided clean water supplies, and designed efficient sewage systems. In a most effective way, they lowered the death rates in societies where endemic and epidemic infectious disease were primary determinants in population control. But while tampering with the death rate, they did nothing with the birth rate. Consequently, many nations developed economic, political, and social problems as a result of overpopulation. As technicians, these HCW were brilliant, successful. As responsible members of the human family, they failed miserably.

Hopefully, we have learned from the past how to frame more appropriate questions than our predecessors. Where they asked "Can malaria be eliminated" or "How can I establish a hospital in the mountains of southeast Asia," we must ask "How can the health of individuals *and* the well-being of this society be improved by my efforts?" Just as germaine is the question, "What are my own personal motivations for involving myself in the health issues of a group to whom I am an outsider?" And most important of all: "What do the inhabitants of this place want?"

The Traditional Healer and the Modern Health Care Worker

Once the former questions are answered—not perfectly, but seriously—the issue still remains: what should be the relationship of the modern HCW with the traditional healer? Perhaps we can address this pressing question more accurately after examining the similarities of both HCW and healer, the differences between them, and the context(s) in which they operate.

The traditional healer and modern HCW share (1) an analogous social role and (2) similar *modus operandi*. They are accorded a special social status and have the social privilege to ask personal questions of patients and touch them in a fashion not accepted in any other kind of interpersonal relationship. They give names to disorders (that is, make "diagnoses"), predict outcomes of disorders (give "prognoses"), and make recommendations regarding treatment.* According to the mutual consent of patient and

---

*From my own experience in Laos, traditional healers—while limited in their therapies—are fairly skilled at diagnosis and prognosis of common disorders. For example, after taking a history and looking at the patient, traditional healers fairly consistently diagnosed "forest fever" (*khai paa*) for the same cases that I—after careful palpation for the the spleen and review of the blood smear—diagnosed "malaria." The same was true of the healers' "dry lung" (*puot heng*) and my "tuber-

healer, treatment may be instituted—or may not be instituted—or a referral made to another treating person. In short, there is a "doctor-patient relationship" of a kind that transcends time, social class, and culture.

The differences have been touched on earlier. Training, world view, evaluation of treatment methods, and sharing of data distinguish the modern HCW from traditional healers. It should be noted, however, that these differences are mostly *intra-professional*. That is, they concern the relationship among healers themselves but do *not* directly concern the healer-patient relationship. While the differences between the traditional healer and modern HCW are certainly of crucial interest to patients and society, nonetheless the *individual* sick and ailing patient desirous of help often does not distinguish between the two—indeed, in many "developing" groups, they initially *cannot* distinguish between the two (Tinling, 1967; Reed *et al*, 1971; Wintrobe, 1973).

This brings us on to the *context* within which modern HCW and traditional healer must function: that is, the patients themselves and the society which they altogether comprise. In the societies which we are discussing, the populace—even though undergoing change—nonetheless have a persistent faith in and expectation of the traditional healer. The same is not initially true of the modern HCW, who is unknown to sick patients and their distraught families. Fortunately for those of us who are modern HCW, patients and their families seem everywhere and always to be basically eclectic in their search for assistance: in the face of dire consequences they are willing to try unproven (i.e. nontraditional) methods of treatment, and in the even of successful treatment they are willing to give the devil his due (Friedson, 1960; Spicer, 1971).

In my experience, a certain historical process evolves in which patients make use of the modern HCW. Briefly stated, the process occurs as follows:

---

culosis" or "lung flukes." Moreover, our prognoses were generally quite similar, though I had the scalpel, the antibiotics, the microscope, and the x-ray machine to make somewhat more specific diagnoses and undertake more specific therapies.

1. Acute trauma, acute infections with fever and signs of sepsis, and superficial tumors are the first to be transferred to the modern HCW. These are the problems in which the HCW has greatest success, and in which the patients and their families can observe the most dramatic results. Initially, only cases are brought which have already received traditional care, but to no avail.

   Many of these patients are close to death when brought by their families. But with intravenous fluids, antibiotics, and fairly simple surgical procedures, most of these patients recover. Such events appear to, the local populace—who know well the face of death since it visits them often—view these recoveries as virtually "miracles." Word spreads rapidly and widely about such events. In a very short time, even the traditional healers refer these cases to the modern HCW (that is, they serve "triage" function by screening patients and sending the most critically ill to the HCW).

2. Chronic and subacute medical problems come to the modern HCW later, and then only after prolonged treatment by numerous traditional healers. Even where the assistance of the modern HCW is sought, patient and family often prefer to continue with the services of traditional healers and the HCW at the same time.

   For example, my friend's minor wife (though his favorite wife) became moribund over a few days with typhoid. Since there was an epidemic of typhoid at the time—and there were deaths by the score—he brought her to the hospital for treatment immediately. After some days on parenteral fluids and antibiotics, it seemed that she might survive. My friend acutely noted, however, that a few patient with his wife's disease died in the hospital even with our "modern" treatment. He was worried. So as to cover all possibilities, he asked if he could bring her home where more lengthy and intensive spirit ceremonies might be performed, yet still arranged for "modern" care. Since she lived less than a kilometer away, I saw no problems in doing my part while the healers did theirs. The patient and family were cheered to have both forms of care at home. (She survived this bout of typhoid.)

3. Psychiatric and psychosomatic cases tend to remain with traditional healers the longest, and do not seek help from the modern HCW except in severe cases (i.e. mutism, suicide attempts, prolonged psychosis). This probably occurs because of (a) loss of communication nuances between the patients and the modern HCW, (b) the frequent success of traditional healers in mild cases, (c) the greater time required by the modern HCW to treat such cases, and (d) the relative naivete

of many modern HCW in the care of such cases—especially in ethnic groups or social classes different from their own.

During my first stay in Laos, I usually referred such patients to a Lao HCW (if one were available) or to a traditional healer. The latter do fairly well with "crisis" or self-limited cases, but not so well with major, chronic, incapacitating disorders. Where a person becomes incapacitated (i.e. unable to work) with such disorders, families often expend huge sums of money going from one traditional healer to another for help.

My point here is that it is primarily the *patient* and the *patient's family* who make the choices regarding whom to consult in the event of health problems. And in cases where traditional healers and modern HCW refer to each other, it is usually to the patient's benefit that the referral is made.

The Issues

For the patient and the patient's family the issue regarding healer and HCW is relatively simple: one uses whatever means available that is most likely to resolve the health problem. For the modern HCW or the politician or the social planner, the matter is not so simple. Collaboration between healer and HCW is not an unmixed blessing; and failure to collaborate has its advantages and disadvantages also. The issues involved include the following:

1. Collaboration by the modern HCW with the traditional healer provides for the psychological comfort of the patient and the family. In itself this conduces to a better therapeutic outcome (i.e. lowered mortality and morbidity). (Jilek, 1971).

2. Good relationships between the modern HCW and the indigenous social system result in earlier and more frequent referrals to the HCW. As this referral relationship proceeds over time, healers often become more adept at referring appropriate cases in an earlier and more treatable phase in the disease. This cooperation enhances health care for the populace (Westermeyer *et al*, 1974).

3. Initially there are not sufficient numbers of modern HCW to displace traditional healers. Thus, a gradual transition from one to the other ordinarily takes place. During this time, the

healer can perform a "triage" function by keeping the less seriously ill and send on major cases to the HCW.

4. Provision of modern health care does *not* just depend on availability of modern HCW (McDermott *et al*, 1972), but also depends on evaluation of a "folk knowledge" among the patient population regarding *how to utilize modern health care*. Evolution of this folk knowledge requires years, and in some ways, decades or even centuries, for a people to acquire.

5. We do not know the effect of collaboration by the modern HCW with the traditional healer on patient behavior. It may have no effect. Or it may enhance the confidence of the patient in the traditional healer. In the latter event, one might argue that as a result (a) effective care by the modern HCW is delayed or even avoided altogether; (b) patients make useless expenditures of money, since the services of traditional healers are often expensive; (c) continued reliance on traditional healers supports magical thinking and an old world view, while needlessly delaying or slowing the turmoil of culture change (Hall and Bourne, 1973).

Once the modern HCW has responded to the political, ethical, and personal questions raised earlier, he or she must address these issues. Even to ignore them is to make a decision, the decision not to collaborate with the traditional healer. Either the *pro* or *contra* decision appears to have some positive and some negative sequelae.

Discussion

In my opinion the "collaborative" approach on the part of the modern HCW is most beneficial for patients and their families; I suspect it may be better for their society. It does not place patients in the conflicted position of having to choose between the two modalities of care. While receiving modern treatment methods that are physiologically beneficial, the patient can receive traditional care that is familiar, reassuring, and psychologically helpful. Moreover, this approach does not precipitate sociocultural discontinuity or anomie experiences. It enables people to place one foot firmly in the familiar past while taking a risky step into the unknown future. In other words, I would argue that the indigenous traditional healer should be gradually displaced by the indigenous modern HCW, until both "traditional" and "modern" healer become one in the same person. Such gradual transitions enhance health, while not having untoward political and economic consequences.

In any event, the role of the traditional healer vis-a-vis the modern HCW in a non-coercive society is determined mostly by patients (i.e. by society at large). Neither traditional healers nor modern HCW have much actual influence over their mutual relationship as it comes into focus in the individual patient. In the main, the patient and the family determine how they will relate to healer and HCW.

Even in coercive societies, the gradual melding of traditional healer and modern HCW into one person has proven most effective. The "barefoot doctor" in China and the "feldsher" in Russia have played major roles in reducing mortality and morbidity. In many areas of the world, the modern trained nurse-midwife has greatly improved maternal and neo-natal health statistics. (Minkowski, 1974; Sidel and Siden, 1974).

In sum, the issue is not so much: traditional healers—to be or not to be? But rather: traditional healers—how gradually should they be replaced by the modern HCW, and how can their social role be most effectively integrated with the knowledge and techniques of the modern HCW?

REFERENCES

Friedson E: "Client control and medical practice," *Amer J Sociology* 65:374-380, 1960.

Haggerty, R.J: "The boundaries of health care," *Pharos*, pp. 106-111, (July) 1972.

Hall, A.L., Bourne, P.G.: "Indigenous therapists in a southern Black urban community, *Archives of General Psychiatry* 28:137-142, 1973.

Jilek, W.G.: "From crazy witch doctor to auxiliary psychotherapist—the changing image of the medicine man," *Psychiatria Clinica* 4:200-220, 1971.

McDermott, W., Deuschle, K.W., Barnett, C.R.: "Health care experiment at Many Farms," *Science* 175:23-31,1972.

Minkowski, A.: "Health care in China and the West," *Hospital*

Practice, pp. 138-146, (July) 1974.

Reed, W.P., Rael, E.D., Hodgin, U.G.: "The cure of plague—two viewpoints," *J. Amer Medical Assoc* 216:1197-1198, 1971

Sidel, V.W., Sidel, R.: "The delivery of medical care in China," *Scientific American* 230: 19-27, 1974.

Spicer, E.H.: "Persistent cultural systems," *Science* 174:795-800, 1971.

Tinling, D. C.: "Voodoo, root work, and medicine," *Psychosomatic Medicine* 29:483-490, 1967.

Westermeyer, J., Tanner, R., Smelker, J.: "Change in health care services for Indian Americans," *Minnesota Medicine* 57:732-735, 1974.

Westermeyer, J.: "Absentee health workers and community participation," *Amer J Public Health* 62: 1364-1369, 1972.

Westermeyer, J., Hausman, W.: "Mental health consultation with government agencies: a comparison of two cases," *Social Psychiatry* 9:137-141, 1974.

UTILIZATION OF PERSISTING CULTURAL VALUES OF MEXICAN-AMERICANS BY WESTERN PRACTITIONERS

Charles Harrison Williams, D.O.

Modern general practitioners have increasingly extended treatment to people of varying cultural backgrounds. In addition to treating organic diseases, practitioners will need to recognize both the functional aspects of organic disease and the therapeutic problems which are purely functional in nature in which no underlying organic cause can be ascertained. Variously, the percentage of functional illness confronting primary care physicians have been estimated from 50 to 80 percent of all presenting complaints. When the cultural frame of reference of the therapist and the client are the same, the labels attached to the medical problems will have the same symbolic significance. Among Mexican-Americans who are the largest single group of Latin Americans in this country estimated at approximately 10 million persons; labels attached to medical entities will be reinterpreted by them to be congruent with existing cultural beliefs and values.

This paper will examine how the Mexican-American developed his cultural frame of reference in relation to his concept of disease and why Mexican folk healing practices or *curanderismo*, as it is known, persists in modern American setting. Finally, the ethical and therapeutic problems of utilizing Mexican-American folk healing concepts and native healers by the western therapist will be considered.

Despite the fact that many Mexican-Americans have been in this country for more than six generations the complex of beliefs and customs associated with *curanderismo* is one of the main traditions persisting in the Mexican-American sub-culture. These customs have persisted in a large part because of the difficulties encountered by these people in becoming a part of the American tradition. In the absence of a new set of assumptions that correspond to conditions as they truly are in his present environment, the Mexican-American is forced to utilize the cultural resources which have always been available or alternatively to develop new institutions within his subculture.

Far from being a homogeneous group, the Mexican-American is composed of peoples who have been acculturating in the American milieu since the early 1800's. Mexican cultural values and frames of reference have been reinforced by the continued close contact with the Mexican society derived from the continued legal and illegal immigration into this country.

The Mexican-Americans' concept of disease differs from the western concept for two reasons. Originally, Mexico was colonized by the Spaniard who conceived of disease based on the Greco-Roman concept of humoral pathology. Disease was based in the ideas that there was a lack of harmony among the various body components which should be cured by nature. This concept of disease was syncretized to the indigenous belief of the Aztecs that illness was the result of sorcery, "evil winds" and non-adherence to the ritual requirements of sacrifices or prayers. These beliefs concerning the origin of disease persisted to the time of the Mexican Independence of 1910. Secondly, with little modification these beliefs were continued under American economic hegemony. While the native Mexican-American had achieved independence from the Spaniard, economic exploitation by the American continued to deprive him of the opportunity of developing the newer western concepts of disease.

When the native Mexican was originally colonized, the Spaniard followed the typical pattern of colonialism by a dominant majority, although they were fewer in number than the subject natives, and an indigenous subordinate minority. Since the dominant majority was fewer in number, the Spaniard co-opted the existing society by removing the ruling minority and replacing them with themselves through force of arms as the new governors, priests, educators and became the ruling elite of the cultural institutions of the native. Thus, superimposed upon the native beliefs, the Spaniard imposed the 15th and 16th century beliefs of religion and medicine. In this manner the socially inferior group, the native, was subjugated and excluded from participation in the ruling society.

American economic colonialism began with the annexation of large parts of the southwest from Spanish colonial rule while extending economic domination over the rest of Mexico, especially in the regime of Porfirio Diaz. Powerful economic interests in the United States, notably agricultural and mining interests, have conspired for economic reasons to manipulate the near bottomless pool of Mexican labor. Treated as an economic asset, the Mexican motivation for naturalization and integration into the American way has been greatly reduced. Such economic exploitation has perpetuated the colonial status of the Mexican-American. He is a minority with cultural and racial characteristics which distinguish him from the majority. This majority generally regard and treat the Mexican minority as inferior and different. Then this minority is excluded from full participation in the society and, therefore, continues to have poorer life chances and fewer rights and less resources. When resources are denied, the minority must fall back upon their own culturally based resources and beliefs. With the absence of adequate educational and economic opportunities folk practices will continue to be utilized as an alternative to the changing and newer medical concepts of disease.

American colonialism has been particularly destructive to the efforts to integrate the native culture with the dominant *Anglo* society. In addition to suppressing the socio-economic opportunities of the Mexican-American minority the functioning social units of the native colonial Mexican were also destroyed, further limiting the resources of the native Mexican American. During the years of Spanish colonialism the functioning unit of the society was the *patron-peon* system. In this system the *patron* assumed the responsibilities and gave direction to the unit. He owned the land, settled disputes, and was the political center for the group. To the *patron* was assigned all of the ruling characteristics of an organized group. In turn, he was responsible to the *peon*. The *peon* looked then to his master for his resources. When the southwest United States was annexed, much of the lands were seized, expropriated, and generally, the *patron-peon* systems were broken down. With the breakdown of the system the poor peasant had no one to replace with a new *patron*. Today the *peon* is essentially a person without a *patron* to whom to turn for aid or resources. As a result the *peon* has had to develop alternate institutions and resources. They had to turn inward among themselves for succor and aid. This process has markedly enhanced the formation and continuance of today's Mexican-American subculture.

Americans have been characterized as aggressive, individually oriented, socially motivated, time conscious and competitive. Also, they have a tendency to forego immediate needs to obtain long term goals or gratifications. These characteristics have been a main theme in American life and have dominated the ethnic and subculture of the immigrating groups. Mexican-American belief systems have been influenced by these characteristics but due to continued immigration from Mexico and the results of continuing American economic colonialism, the Mexican-American subculture has a vastly different orientation.

Running through the Mexican culture are two great themes: family and religion. To understand Mexican-Americans is to know the family relationships and the religious beliefs. Mexican family life is based upon two propositions: (1) the unquestionable and absolute supremacy of the father and; (2) the necessary and absolute sacrifice of the mother. After marriage the wife usually lives with the husband's parents for some years. Males in a Mexican-American family are encouraged to develop *Machismo*, that is, to exhibit the qualities of virility, courage and manliness. They also look to the family for support and help in times of stress. On the other hand, the wife is expected to be wife, mother and subservient to the dominant males in the household. She becomes the center of the home and her whole social sphere will revolve around her children and other female relatives in the family.

Religion, the second great theme among Mexican-American families is professed to be Catholicism. However, Catholicism varies from orthodox Catholicism in the upper socio-economic group, to folk Catholicism in the middle and lower socio-economic groups. Folk Catholicism is syncretized from the gods and religious practices of the indigenous races present before the Spanish conquest and from the 15th and 16th century Catholicism introduced by the Iberian conquerors. Today, in most Mexican homes, religion is physically visible at the family altar and consists of a table of holy images, cnadles, pictures of the family, holy water and an incense burner. Festooned on the walls will be numerous scapulars, medals and religious adornments. The Mexican feels and sees God all about him. He considers himself to be of little importance in the universe and that his fate is decided for him before birth, and since God sent him he will have to leave when God calls him. Acceptance and appreciation of things as they are has led to a present and fatalistic outlook for the Mexican-American—an orientation that is quite incompatable with the futuristic orientated *Anglo* culture.

A *curandero*, or folk healer, may be anyone in the family or community. Usually, a healer is a regularly employed person in the community who seems, additionally, to possess the abilities to heal or to help. Also, the healer will be a very religious person and exemplify all the virtues and values considered important to the Mexican-American. He is basically an unselfish person and recognizes that God is the ultimate source of all well being. The *curandero* and his patients recognize that disease and suffering can befall any man but they are always concerned as to why this disease occurs at this time and why it should appear in this man. Thus, all disease is presented in a social context, for in addition to curing the disease there must be an attempt at relief of social conflict with the end result of reintegration of the patient into his society. Such reconciliation must also be socially acceptable to the community and his family.

A *curandero* or other native folk healer enjoys great respect and status among the subculture. In order to understand how he could develop respect and apparent effectiveness utilizing a deficient and erroneous concept of disease and dispensing relatively innocuous medications, such as herbs and teas and, in many instances, little more than holy water, we will have to examine the sources of success for all therapists. In general, we have broadly categorized medicine into two general areas, one, that of organic disease with its objective manifestations and two, functional or mental diseases char-

112

acterized by subjective complaints. Whether the presenting complaint of a patient is either organic or functional, all western therapists are familiar with the inherent mechanism within the human body which will cause spontaneous cures. In fact, most complaints will subside regardless of the treatment rendered by a therapist and when the complaint is apparently healed by the ministrations of the therapist, both the client and therapist will attribute the cure to the healer. Healers are able to attribute to themselves both the cures which he might actually himself effect and also those which would spontaneously occur regardless of the ministrations of the healer. Obviously the *curandero* is successful if for no more reason than that he is credited for organic cures which would occur as a result of the normally functioning defense mechanisms of the human organism. Secondly, in the broad area of functional or mental diseases the *curandero* is treating the client within the same cultural frame of reference. Most functional diseases are an abnormal response to the society in which they live. There may be conflict within the society between its members or value conflicts within the belief system of a member. Perhaps a taboo has been broken, a family argument, abnormal role behavior, or possibly other socially unacceptable behavior has occurred. Within these settings the *curandero* or native healer will attempt a cure based on the common cultural and societal beliefs. When viewed in this context the *curandero* approaches the success rate of the western therapist in organic disease, and in treating the functional problems, may be more effective with the native Mexican-American than the western therapist since the client-therapist may have similar cultural beliefs and orientations and is able to obtain once again a high cure rate.

Mexican cultural beliefs and orientation were carried with Mexican-Americans who began to immigrate to the northern part of the United States from the southwest beginning during World War II and continuing during the Korean conflict. Due to the labor shortage in industry and agriculture when the war effort reached its maximum, Mexican-Americans were encouraged by the prospects of socio-economic opportunity to enter the northern labor pool. As is common with many ethnic groups, the Mexican-Americans tended to develop enclaves and communities. They were united by a common language, cultural beliefs and values, all of which differed from the indigenous *Anglo* population.

In southeastern Michigan two large populations have developed. One, on the lower southwest side of Detroit and the other an area concentrated on the southeast side of Pontiac, near the center of the city. Almost all of the Mexican-Americans are employed today in the industrial sector of the economy, principally, the automobile industry. Unions have been instrumental in providing job security. In the agricultural sector there was no such protection and most have left agriculture for employment in the factories, for in agriculture they were exposed to the same economic and job discrimination they knew from their job experiences in the southwest.

Today's Mexican-American presents a full range of cultural beliefs and values ranging from those of the old native Mexican culture to the values and beliefs of the American society. Within this broad diversity there tends to be two broad categories.

One group tends to be composed of the older original emigres and the subsequent ones who have been emigrating over the succeeding years. This group more nearly approximates the values and beliefs of the Mexican and southwest Mexican-American culture. In some instances many members of this group are still unable to communicate in English. This burden has fallen heaviest on the mother, since the father goes to work and assimilates English from his co-workers while the children attend school where normally only English is taught. Since the mother is thus isolated from the American community her friends will, of necessity, be other Spanish speaking people. Situations of this nature tend to reinforce and confirm the old native beliefs and lend mistrust to the American belief system which they do not understand and have little opportunity to learn. In health matters they will turn to friends or relatives for advice before seeking out western physicians.

The other broad category of Mexican-Americans is basically the generation born in the north and who have received their education from the American school system. They have been exposed to American cultural values over a long period of time and some develop belief systems approaching the American, however, rarely is a Mexican-American encountered even today that is really *anglicized*. It seems there is always a lingering attachment to the old Mexican-American customs. Most noticeable of the differences between the two groups is the behavior of the females. Women of the anglicized group work in factories, restaurants, as secretaries, and in general have had considerably more education. Contrast this with the older women who almost never work outside the home and received little or no formal education. Perhaps they might be employed to perform household chores in another home or, with the entire family obtain agricultural work such as picking beans, peas, fruit or thinning beets on a seasonal basis—jobs in which today's younger woman will not participate. Another striking feature between the groups is the freedom of the younger females. Traditionally, the women would find entertainment among themselves by attending a movie, bingo or visiting with each other within the home setting. Older women will be seen with their husbands at family functions or close community functions especially when these are church oriented. On the other hand, the younger women are attending mixed functions, dating, bowling, entering clubs and generally enjoying the freedoms similar to the younger American women. When the younger women marry and form new family units they have tended to move into the American community by breaking or loosening the tradition of close family relationships characteristic of Mexican families. With the changing family relationship there has been a marked increase in divorce and desertion by the husband and in illegitimacy. In the older Mexican community this would be extremely rare behavior. Interestingly, this behavior has become more commonplace as the socio-economic opportunities have increased. When the Mexican-American was in the poverty situation, the families were close knit and dependent on one another and divorce and desertion were almost non-existent.

With the increased affluence provided by their industrial jobs in the form of prepaid insurance, required immunization programs in the schools and an increasing assimilation of western culture, the Mexican-American is presenting himself more often to *Anglo* practitioners for help. The following cases will present some of the problems of the amalgam of native with western beliefs in the care of Mexican-Americans.

Case 1. Mrs. O.G., a 23-year-old Mexican-American woman was first seen by me because she would have violent episodes of temper. During the last episode she had tried to attack her husband with a knife. She also had recurring spells of crying and often felt like she was going to "blow up" or explode. She was concerned that in one of the spells she would injure one of her children. She denied any conflict with her husband and, in fact, since moving from Texas the family situation has improved financially. She did state that she was having trouble getting to sleep. She also had some shaking spells and had considerable, as she described, "shaking inside." She denied any previous serious illnesses. Physical examination revealed no organic problems. Although there was a small cross tatooed on her chest of which she admitted shame and was quite reluctant to show me, she stated that it had been present all her life and did not understand its significance. She and her family had recently emigrated from a small south Texas town to Pontiac, Michigan, where her husband had found employment in one of the automobile plants. She was the youngest of 15 children. However, on history obtained later from her brother, she is actually the illegitimate daughter of the oldest sister. She was reared by her grandparents, whom she considered her parents. She was married at 16, which she maintains was normal at that time in Texas. She has had three children.

It was felt she was reacting to the stress of the long move from Texas and to the separation from her family. In the Mexican context, the family unit is very strong and one looks to various members for support. In Michigan she had only one friend with whom to talk or discuss problems. She was diagnosed as acute anxiety with periods of depression, basically a functional problem. She was placed on a therapy of trifluoperazine to relieve the anxiety and to normalize her sleep habits. She was encouraged to develop close friendships and, additionally, a brother was encouraged to move from Texas to the Pontiac area. To further help the patient and her husband understand her problems, I explained that in their Mexican-American culture they characterize this condition as *susto*. In the Mexican-American culture this means "emotional fright" and is usually the result of some traumatic experience. The patient was aware of the term *susto* and was able to better conceptualize her problem. The use of the terms anxiety and depression were not meaningful. As a result of her understanding, use of tranquilizers and a re-socialization in the Pontiac community she adequately coped with her problems and over the three years she was under treatment she was able to function satisfactorily in her new environment.

Case 2. A.R., an eight-month-old Mexican-American infant was brought to the hospital emergency room. History obtained revealed that he had been sick about a week; and that he had begun with temperature elevations, some vomiting and a severe diarrhea. After 2-3 days, he improved but the day before admittance had rapidly worsened, and was now vomiting as well as having a severe diarrhea. Physical examination of the baby revealed a lethargic, well developed male with a temperature of 104^6. The tongue surface was coated and furry. The skin was dry and wrinkled easily when pinched as a result of the loss of normal skin elasticity. The eyes were sunken and the anterior fontanelle was depressed. It was felt the child had severe gastroenterititis with dehydration although the possibility of other more severe conditions such as epidemic diarrhea, meningitis or food poisoning would need to be entertained. Need for hospitalization was explained to the family. There was resistance by the family to leaving the baby and asked if an injection or medicine would be adequate so they could take the baby with them. It was explained that since the soft spot at the top of the head was depressed this represented a serious loss of fluids and since he still had vomiting and a severe diarrhea, fluids would have to be replaced by intravenous therapy. Also, I explained that Mexican-Americans sometimes call the sunken fontanelle *caida de la mollera*. Our treatment would be to replace

117

fluids until the fontanelle was no longer sunken. When the disease was explained in Mexican folk terminology, the father said the grandmother had made this diagnosis and had tried to correct the sunken fontanelle by pushing up on the palate and giving an herb tea. At first her treatment seemed to be satisfactory, however, when the baby worsened, the family brought the baby to the hospital. I explained that the tea as a fluid replacement was a good attempt to help with fluids but that pressure on the palate would not be useful. Replacement fluid therapy quickly alleviated the dehydration and the child was sent home with the parents in 2-3 days.

Case 3. Mrs. M.S. age 28, divorced, has had two children and two abortions and then had missed two menstrual periods and was afraid she might be pregnant again. She had been taking birth control pills regularly. Her pregnancy test and abdominal examinations were negative for pregnancy. She was told that it was doubtful that she was pregnant. She has had two abortions and they were very emotionally upsetting to her. She appeared doubtful that the cause of her amenorrhea could be due to the birth control pills. However, she agreed to return in a month if she remained amenorrheic. In the meantime a request was received from social services for aid in a pregnancy for this woman. When she reappeared still without menstruating and, again, the pregnancy tests were normal and the physical examination revealed a normal sized uterus, her therapy was changed to promote a normal menstrual period utilizing a different complex of hormones. After her next menstruation I asked her why she was so adamant in maintaining the possibility of pregnancy. She felt that she was either pregnant or *embrujada*, that is, hexed or bewitched. Since her divorce there had been considerable conflict between her ex-husband's parents and herself over the children, especially since she had taken them to her parents' home to live. When she failed to menstruate she was afraid the father's parents were causing her to be ill so she continued to hope she was pregnant. When she menstruated she was relieved of both fears, i.e. that of unwanted pregnancy and relief from the possibility of being *embrujada* (bewitched) by the childrens' paternal grandparents.

One of the main objectives in a therapist-client relationship is the necessity for the therapist to name or to label the health problem. To label a hitherto unknown medical problem is to relieve anxiety by giving meaning and understanding to a series of previously unexplained phenomena. Since most western therapists are of American origin, the difficulty is apparent when trying to be effective in a distant socio-cultural setting. Too often the western therapist will simply ignore the cultural interpretations of the client's disease and apply the interpretation from his (the therapist's) scientific western frame of reference. In the cases illustrated, it was necessary to reinterpret the therapist's scientific frame of reference to the patient's cultural frame of reference. All of the cases, whether purely functional or organic, contained a native folk component that when recognized and shared with the patient increased rapport and communication, relieved anxiety and enhanced the therapeutic setting. Since folk traditions and modern healing have existed side by side even in the most modern of societies, for the therapist to be ignorant of, or unaware of, the traditional beliefs of his client is to leave unexplored certain avenues to fuller understanding of the total patient. Rarely will the patient of a subordinate culture reveal beliefs and feelings to a therapist of the more dominant culture. When treating patients with different cultural backgrounds the western therapist will need to initiate explorations into the social and cultural feelings and beliefs of the client. An understanding and knowledge of the folk beliefs increase the empathy of the therapist, gives dignity to the beliefs of the subcultural group and enhances the therapist-client relationship.

Ethical considerations of utilizing the *curandero* (native healer) need to be explored. Certainly to send a patient directly to a traditional healer for help and discharge them from your care could be construed as associating with cults, quackery or associating with unlicensed practitioners. On the other hand, when one considers that the very characteristics of the *curandero* reflect the best in ideals and values of the Mexican society it would seem that to maintain rigid ethical considerations would constitute a real barrier to obtaining relevant help for some clients. Perhaps if the *curanderos* were utilized somewhat as western therapists utilize clergymen, marriage counselors, social workers and the like there would be little ethical problems. One immediate problem is the relative lack of true *curanderos* but the presence of many neighborhood healers. Most of these healers are employed at other jobs and often have little education. Another consideration is that many clients will have had previous consultation with the neighborhood healer before seeking a western physician or in some instances be simultaneously consulting with the native healer at the same time he is under treatment by a western physician.

Probably the preferable ethical method for western physicians would be to hire native healers to aid in the therapy while the western physician supervises the total therapy. Since the native healer treats all diseases, both functional and organic, as a social disease the western physician will need to consider and treat organic ailments and to prescribe necessary medication for both the functional and organic entities. In this context the *curandero* would be available to help in obtaining adequate history, interpreting the health beliefs of the client and giving suggestions for relief of the social conflicts. Another point worthy of consideration is the difference in approach to the client by the western trained therapist as contrasted by the approach by the traditional Mexican-American folk healer. Western therapists devise therapies on a direct therapist-client basis or to group clients with similar appearing complaints into therapy sessions. Contrast this to the *curandero* who invariably works with the client and his family as the group. Many times the therapy is conducted in the client's normal home environment and where large parts of the therapy involve the family members. In this respect he would be functioning as a family therapist. This approach is similar to modern psychiatric thinking that therapy for mental illnesses is perhaps best treated in the client's normal environment rather than to remove him to some institutional setting that is foreign to the societal environment where he is to eventually live. Objectives of treatment will be more nearly realized if the client can be socially and mentally reintegrated into the environment in which he must function.

Our experience has been that we are able to be very

effective in organic disease. There is a growing awareness among the younger Mexican-Americans that the western therapist is more effective in organic disease than the native healer. Many times we see far advanced infectious diseases or other medical problems which have probably been treated by the family or neighborhood healers prior to consultation with western therapists. When treating functional problems the lack of a similar cultural frame of reference add immeasurably to the difficulty of successfully treating socially derived complaints. Rarely will minority patients offer information of a cultural nature to a western physician. These efforts must be initiated by the physician. Many times the needed information can be obtained from other members of the family.

Whether the therapist today is treating members of his own culture or of very different ethnic and cultural background, the therapist to be increasingly effective, will need to be aware that the cultural frames of reference between the therapist and client may be different. This is significant because in different cultures the labels, symbols and values of the culture are interpreted differently. Knowledge that there is reinterpretation of similar labels removes one area of sociocultural conflict and gives greater significance to the therapist-client relationship. Therapy of a member of a different background may require some method of consultation with a traditional healer to help obtain history and aid in interpreting underlying folk beliefs as well as functioning as a family therapist. Rapport between therapist and client will be enhanced and therapy will have been given greater opportunities for success.

NOTES

1Biesanz, Mavis Heltunen and Biesanz, John, *Introduction to Sociology*. New Jersey:Prentice-Hall, Inc., 1973.

2Clark, Margaret. *Health in the Mexican American Culture*. Berkeley: University of California Press, 1970.

3Keiv, Ari, *Curanderism: Mexican American Folk Psychiatry*. New York: The Free Press, 1968.

4Lewis, Oscar, "Husbands and Wives in a Mexican Village: a study of Role Conflict," *American Anthropologist.* Vol. LI, No. 1 (Oct-Dec 1949) p. 602-610.

[5]Moore, Joan. "Colonialism: The Care of the Mexican Americans" in *Nation of Nations: The Ethnic Experiences and the Racial Crises.* Rose, Peter I., Ed., New York: Random House, 1912.

[6]Modern, William, *The Mexican American of South Texas.* New York: Holt, Rhinehart and Winston, 1965.

[7]Toor, Frances, *A Treasury of Mexican Folkways.* New York: Crown Publishers, 1947.

THE IMPACT OF COLONIALISM ON AFRICAN CULTURAL HERITAGE WITH SPECIAL REFERENCE TO THE PRACTICE OF HERBALISM IN NIGERIA

Chief J. O. Lambo

The evils done to the Natural and Cultural heritage by the insatiable Colonial Masters in the name of Civilisation in Africa in the past are only now beginning to appear in the world scientific literatures. This is because during the age of suppression, no writer will be bold and courageous enough to describe in black and white the atrocities done by the Colonial Masters to the African's cultural heritage.

Science owes a big debt to the people of Africa, for the basis of scientific development was supplied by the African cultures. It may be said without fear of exaggeration that the past historians have devoted much less efforts and talent to this important aspect of Colonial impact on African cultures. Only detailed, painstaking investigation in which African researchers themselves are to play a major part, will provide the groundwork for recreating a panorama of African's past and thus reviewing the lost African cultural heritage. Many of the lost propositions, and culture in the field of Therapy and Art will most likely be amplified, supplemented and interpreted in a modern way by the joint efforts of African researchers. But it should be undertaken in a close unity with the study of modern problems.

The student of African contemporary history faces many difficulties in revealing the atrocities done by the Colonial Masters to African cultures, because there was no written record. Evidence was only taken from the traces left behind and the oral history given by some old people. The revival was made possible when the political situation on the continent was changed, and the people began to taste the sweetness of independence and having a sense of responsibility. As the subject matter in this volume is the impact of Colonialism on African culture, references must be made to the activities of the British, the French, the Portuguese, the Germans and the Spanish in dividing the continent among themselves in which the British took the lion's share. It will also be of interest to know what has brought these people to

123

the continent of Africa, and the motives behind the suppression of African cultures in many fields.

Industrial Revolution

In a precis form, industrial revolution means a movement which quickly brings about a change in the nature of industry, and necessitated expansion in trade. Around the eighteenth century, there was an industrial revolution in England, which marked a period of transition from ancient to modern method of industry. This period of transition, though gradual, brought about outstanding increases in production resulting in the desire to find new places for exportation and the search for raw materials. The revolution in industry and agriculture resulted not only in new methods but also brought about a new way of life, and alteration in the standard of living.

The English people before this period were largely rural, concerned only with local materials, within their own country. With the growth of industry, they now form an industrial community and had the desire to trade all over the world. The industrial manual processes were replaced by machines and thus resulted in the increase of production and reduction in manual labour which again brought about unemployment. Thus, these conditions, that is, increase in production and unemployment and many other factors necessitated the desire to colonise some places. At the beginning of the period of revolution, the bulk of the raw materials were locally obtained, but as production increased, these sources of supply became inadequate and England had to find other sources of supply. At this time the colonisation of Africa and South America were paramount in their minds. This was further heightened by the rise in the population which accompanied the industrial revolution and led to more food being required by the people. By this time every European nation of importance was eager to improve its trade resources at the expense of every other nation and their target was Africa.

Exploration

Another important factor, which brought the Europeans into Africa especially the Western part, was the slave trade. Terrible though the slave trade was, it was through that trade that the inhabitant of West Africa first acquired the products of Britain and other European countries. Slaves were bartered for goods produced by British factories. The cessation of traffic in human beings did not check the desire of the inhabitants for the imported goods and thus it came about that legitimate trade was thus established. This gave strong footing to this destroyer of African cultures. The first important journey of discovery in West Africa was made by Mungo Park. This young Scottish doctor was employed by an Association composed of persons interested in Africa and its geography.

In the year 1822 an expedition was set out under the leadership of Dr. Oudney, organised by the British Government. Oudney was accompanied by two men, a Naval officer named Clapperton and an Army officer named Denham. After a preliminary journey into the Sahara, Lake Chad was reached in 1823 after which Bornu, a city in Nigeria, was traversed and Kano was visited. Though Oudney died at Kano, Clapperton continued with the exploration of Nigeria. This was the beginning of the destruction of the cultural heritage and suppression of natural powers as practised by the indigenous people. A similar route was followed in 1825 and 1826 by Major Laing, a Scotsman in the British Army, who crossed the Sahara from Tripoli. Others were Richard and John Lander. These were among the people who paved the way for the British government to establish its authority by colonising the country and destroying the cultural heritage of the people.

The Religion

Another important weapon used by the Colonial masters to destroy the cultural heritage was religion. The missionaries came to Nigeria around the fifteenth century and professed

125

that their main duty would be to educate the people and render some medical services. These religious bodies had been inspired by David Livingstone, that famous missionary explorer of Central Africa, who said among other things:— "In the glow of love which Christianity inspires, I resolved to devote my life to the alleviation of human misery." And in this continent of Africa, indeed, there was plenty of human misery for missionaries to endeavor to alleviate. There was the misery resulting from sickness, the misery of the slave trade, the misery caused by fear of such things as human sacrifice and child-stealing, and the results of superstitious beliefs of various forms, such as those which led to the common practice of murder of twins. With these inspiring words, many people joined the band and a host of missionaries bombarded the continent of Africa. Besides the British, the Portuguese were the first Europeans to explore the West Coast of Africa. In 1447, they reached the River Gambia and in 1742, a Portuguese called Fernao Dapo reached Lagos. These Portuguese explorers were not merely traders or religious persons, but they were in search of power. They wanted to form alliances with local Kings, militarily and economically, in order that they might have a strong footing. Another distinguished person who served on the west coasts of Africa was Thomas Birth Freeman, a half caste, who was born in 1809 at a place near Winchester, Hampshire, England.

Freeman came from England with several new missionaries. These missionaries did not limit their activity with the preaching of Christianity but waged war on things Native. In the field of therapy, they branded the Herbalists as witch doctors and their method of healing as rural, unscientific and unhygenic. The Metaphysicians were regarded as pagans, idol worshippers, superstitious and barbaric. Thus they gradually changed the mentality of the majority of people. Those who have the full knowledge of African science, began to forsake them in the interest of religion. The sick began to run away from the Herbalists and those who know the ability of the Herbalists in the field of Therapy would go to them at night. The inspired Idols worshiped by the people were broken. The works of art were destroyed. Synthetic medicine replaced the natural drugs and the people did not take any trouble to find out and compare the efficacy of the two methods.

The Practice of Herbalism

The practice of Herbalism was carried out in all civilised countries before the introduction of synthetic medicine. In the early Middle Ages, physicians used many herbs for the medicines. This follows the great classical works of Hippocrates (460-377 B.C.). Also Galen (130-200 A.D.) introduced the use of many herbs. It was about the time of the Reformation (1493-1541 A.D.) that Paracelsus introduced the use of mineral drugs. In England, the Royal College of Physicians obtained letter of patents in 1518, during the reign of Henry VIII (1491-1547) with powers similar to those now possessed by the General Medical Council. But at the same time, an act of parliament was passed whereby anyone having a knowledge of the healing properties of herbs was allowed to make use of such knowledge. This was the beginning of the practice of herbalism in all civilised countries. Herbalism spread to America with the Pilgrim Fathers and a rather distinctive set of plants came into use. Many of these were taken from the Red Indians. It was Samuel Thomson who introduced them in the year 1769-1843. Since then, the practice of herbalism has been in progress with great success. Despite all these facts, the missionaries intensified their activities to destroy everything native. The motive behind all these was to wipe out completely all indigenous *powers* and African Science, so that God the father (Government) might find it easy to acquire and colonise many countries in Africa with no fear of opposition or resistance.

The Government

At first, four British firms were trading in Nigeria, which later became the Royal Niger Company around the year 1977 at the persuasion of Captain George Coldie Taubman, an officer of the British Army, who later became a trader. This company did not concentrate on trade alone but exercised a bit of force to govern the natives. When the Royal Niger Company tried to expand its administration, it met with great difficulty, for even though Royal in name, it could hardly be expected to negotiate directly with the representatives of other European countries. Thus the British Government was invited and was represented by Lord Aberdare and Sir George Goldie. This move brought many West African countries under the British rule as protectorates. In the year 1861, because of the intensity of inter-tribal war, Lagos which was the capital of Nigeria was ceded to the British Government so that she might be protected against invaders. Later the British rule was extended into the interior of the country and thus the whole of Nigeria became a British Protectorate.

Now the aspiration of the missionaries to wipe out all things native was backed up by the force of law. All herbal preparations were regarded as criminal juju. The people became westernised with a Colonial mentality. Those who wore native dresses were regarded as illiterates and un-educated. Those who ate native foods were regarded as poor, under fed and diseased. Many churches were established and the people were induced to throw away all their herbal remedies as such materials were contrary to the laws of God. The power of Invisibility, Soul Projection, Airy Movement, Soul Transference, and effective words for curative purposes, were completely destroyed in the name of Christianity. Pregnant women, who experienced difficulty at labor were heavily blamed by the nurses because they suspected that they had gone to the homes of herbalists, hence the trouble at labor.

Death should not occur in the dispensary of herbalists. If it happened, the herbalist would be convicted for administering poison that killed the patient. This state of affairs continued and the herbalists as a whole became very poor, relegated to the background and regarded as inferior. They hardly could get wife to marry. In fairness, they tackled all the most difficult cases that the so-called modern doctors termed hopeless. The orthodox doctors quickly seized the opportunity and charged exhorbitantly for the little service they rendered to the patients. They engaged in sinister campaigns against the herbalists, though they realised fully that much could be gotten from herbs. There were some ingredients, which should not be used or touched by the herbalists, on the point that they were dangerous. These included live lizards, chameleons, parts of human beings, etc. For little mistakes made by the herbalist, all his herbal medicine would be taken away to the so-called "government analyst" who knew nothing about the practice of herbalism. The tremendous amount of works done by the herbalists in the field of health services in the country were ignored. It was evident that the few orthodox doctors concentrated in the towns and cities, whereas the people in these areas were not more than four per cent of the whole population. The remaining ninety-six per cent depended mainly on the herbalists for their health care. The main arguments of the detractors were that the herbalists have no standard dosage, they could not diagnose diseases, their laboratories were filthy, they were not trained, etc. These arguments were vague, untenable, unreasonable and devoid of all elements of truth. The herbalists knew well what they were doing; the knowledge was inherited from their fathers and grandfathers, coupled with keen observation and practical experience. They have the full knowledge of the therapeutic virtues of herbs and they were in full control of their uses. Thus there were two distinct groups of professionals: the orthodox medical practitioners who were the real beneficiaries of the white man's colonial rule and the indigenous herbal medical practitioners who were the silent majority for whom the British colonial rule was a negation of all they held dear in the indigenous realm.

Crusade of Emancipation

The crusade of emancipation from the yoke of imperialism so far as natural and cultural heritage is concerned, began in the middle forties. By that time, an economist, who hailed from the Eastern part of Nigeria, by name Mbonu Ojike, started a campaign against all foreign goods. His key words were "Boycott the Boycottable." This campaign nearly changed completely the social outlook of the people. Foreign dress, foods and fashions were boycotted. Agitation for internal autonomy and complete independence began. The colonial masters became restless, they employed all sorts of weapons at their command to fight the agitators. Laws of sedition came into being, there were mass imprisonments, detention, imposition of heavy fines, etc. Regardless of all these atrocities, the nationalists were on the increase and the impact of colonialism was fading little by little, while colonial mentality was giving way to patriotic ideas.

In the field of therapy, the orthodox medical practitioners continued their war of detraction on herbal drugs with unabated intensity, until the year 1947, when the Nigerian Association of Medical Herbalists came into being. The formation of the Association was brought about by a strange circumstance. It happened that a daughter of one herbalist swallowed a coin. She was taken to the hospital where she was X-rayed, the expatriate Senior Medical Officer in charge told the herbalist that his daughter would have to go through an operation. The herbalist rejected this suggestion and took his daughter home. He administered an herbal purgative. The girl stooled the coin the next day. He took the stool with the coin to the Senior Medical Officer, who was surprised and advised the formation of the Association for the improvement of herbal practice in Nigeria. Thus the Herbalist Association was inaugurated.

The Association after being led by two men in succession, came under the control of one dynamic young man, who happened to be an educationist and was in his early thirties, who became President of the Association. His name was Chief Joseph Olusola Lambo. He was convinced about the efficacy of herbal drugs for he was once a beneficiary of herbal medicine. He started the crusade of emancipation with zeal and vigor. He was very vivid in his remarks about the efficacy of herbal drugs and he used all necessary information media to disseminate his doctrine. Government was called upon to institute Research Centres for the investigation of the properties of herbs. In the middle fifties, a hearing was given by the Federal Government to this call. The sum of eighteen thousand pounds (about $54,000) was allocated for research into the properties and potentialities of herbs at the University of Ibadan, which was the oldest University in Nigeria. Thus, the search for therapeutic virtues of herbs began. The method used, of course, was not devoid of colonial mentality, for the herbalists who were in command of the knowledge were not consulted. The pharmacists would get a single leaf, put it in a bottle of acid and observe the reactions. To an herbalist, this was a barren exercise for no useful extraction could be made from such a method.

In course of time, other universities were established and the Department of Pharmacognosy was set up in each of the Universities and a more vigourous research work was conducted. The most conspicuous person among the researchers was a young, dynamic, and energetic doctor of the Department of Chemistry and the School of Mathematical and Physical Sciences called Professor E.A. Akisanya, a Ph.D. and a researcher at the University of Lagos. It was through his efforts that the practice of herbalism came into the limelight. He organised an International Symposium on Traditional Therapy in December 1973, to which many international figures attended. The discussions from this historic Symposium earned the herbalists much credit, for the generality of the people began to realise the importance of herbal drugs. A similar Symposium on Medicinal Plants followed at the University of Ife in April 1974 and another one was scheduled to take place in Cairo in July 1975. Thus the practice of herbalism became the concern of the whole world. The herbalists were now consulted and a joint consultative committee was formed. At a conference in Africa, the Director General of the World Health Organisation made a pronouncement that the time has now come, when traditional medicine should be examined and analysed for the purpose of mass production of herbal remedies. A similar call was made by the Deputy Director General of the World Health Organisation, Professor T. A. Lambo.

This inspiration stimulated the activities of the Pharmacognosists in their research works. The extractions of active principle of many plants continue in many universities and some of the virtues discovered are antibiotic. Still the

131

pharmacists contend that the method of extraction cannot ensure protection of drugs in commercial quality. Instead, they argue that the drugs produced by the herbalists should have been examined, tasted and preserved. At this juncture, I will devote some paragraphs to the description of the healing powers of herbs as given by the herbalists themselves.

The Healing Powers of Herbs

It has been claimed by the herbalists that herbal remedies are unsurpassed in their efficacy and in their complete safety in use as curative drugs. The drugs are the salvation of many chronic cases which have been termed hopeless by the modern doctors. The herbal drugs are rich in minerals, vitamins and other micro-nutrients which enable the body to manufacture when required all the substances necessary to combat disease in all its forms and manifestations. Without these vital substances the cell structures of the body may not be able to combat the armies of infections which beset them. These micro-nutrients which are found in herbs give the body the means to cure and also help to maintain healthy cell structure and thus prevent disease. Herbs are natural and they contain a variety of substances in organic combination and in the proportion compatible with the human body. They are easily assimilable and readily available as therapeutic agents in the body. Though herbal drugs will not quickly suppress pain as some pills do, yet they have a far more beneficial and constructive effect on the body. Many herbs have cleansing effect and they are almost in the majority. There are many others for other needs. There are herbs for each bodily disease. All parts of herbs are used, medicinally, e.g. the leaves, flowers, bark, root, juice, and even the seeds. They are made in form of decoction, powder, lotion, ointment, according to circumstances and needs.

The number of remedies obtained from plants was in the increase. This followed the result of researches which showed that many powerful active agents are stored in plants. Through physiological and biochemical researches, it may be possible to grow new and better varieties of medicinal plants with higher yield of active substances. In future the production of plant materials and the medicinal preparations obtained from them will be in sufficient quantity. Active substances for various diseases are readily available in plants and their potency is excellent. It has been shown through researches that a single leaf may contain more than one property in certain proportion and that one herb may cure more than one disease. Bamboo, which is in the grass family, is said to contain one valuable mineral salt called silica. This mineral salt performs wonderful works in the body, it has been termed nature's surgeon. Where there is pus to be discharged such as boils, abscesses, carbuncles, etc. this salt is indicated. It will bring about the discharge of the pus. Lack of silica may cause inability to connect one's thoughts, bad memory and nervous disorders. Other herbs are:

1. *Fungi*: This is an out-growth, at times they can be found on rotten plants, or on living plants as a parasite. In some places, they come directly from the soil. They are mostly white in color and round like an umbrella. It was from this simple herbal out-growth that the remarkable anti-biotic drug—penicillin was made. This drug is an organic substitute for some dangerous chemical drugs and it is highly efficacious in the treatment of venereal diseases. The powder made from fungus is an excellent remedy against itch, yaws, nettle-rash and other skin diseases. This herb is also used for pregnant women to facilitate easy delivery.

2. *African Cinchona*: This herb is mainly used against fever, gout, rheumatism, rise in temperature, headache and other inflammatory conditions. It is a very popular herb in Africa and is often used as medicine.

3. *Mahogany Bark*: The drug made from this herb is an excellent remedy for anaemia, amenorrhea and other blood diseases. It is an excellent tonic. When it is fresh, it has some odor. The leaves are sometimes used. It contains certain oil, and an ointment is sometimes made out of it for rubbing sprains and bruises. The infusion from this herb is just like wine. When potash is added, it causes the free flow of menstrual period and makes it become clean and brightly colored. With other ingredients it cures strokes or paralysis.

The essence is better released when the herb is cooked and allowed to brew for some time. For stroke or paralysis, a cold concoction of it is made and the patient uses the water to bathe. It is also used for hypertension or nervousness.

4. *Red Raspberry*: This herb is very rich in alkaline and drug made from it is used for most of the feminine complaints. Among its many uses is to reduce pain for a pregnant woman who is about to deliver. Tea made from this herb gives strength to a woman after birth. It also increases the flow of breast milk. It has a cleansing power by acting on the womb. It is perfectly safe to take at all times. When it is mixed with other ingredients, it prevents miscarriage. It is also used as a douche against leucorrhea and other feminine discharges. It is an excellent remedy for excessive bleeding. Raspberry has been used successfully in all feminine troubles, diarrhoea, dysentery, cholera, vomiting of women when they are pregnant.

5. *Traculia Africana*: This herb is most remarkable in the treatment of convulsion, giddiness, vertigo, shaking of the arms and legs and sometimes the head. It cures epilepsy when mixed with other ingredients. It is an excellent remedy for those who are excitable. It is very useful in the treatment of delirium, caused by heavy drinking. It is the root that is most used and the common method is to make an infusion of it. It is used for small children as a preventive against convulsion or other nervous manifestations as might have been developed before birth, if the mother is not well treated. It is suppressive in its effect and it is used for pregnant women, when the pregnancy is about six months old. This is just to ensure that during labor, the women may not experience vertigo as the result of loss of blood.

With these few descriptions of the healing properties of herbs, it could be seen that if proper research is carried out, many wonderful drugs will be produced that will fill the gap created by inadequacy of synthetic drugs and also free the patients from iatrogenic diseases. But in order to bring the practice of herbalism on the proper footing and supply the health needs of many patients in the rural areas, the herbalists should be aided to modernise their system. This assistance may come from the government or any charitable organisation. The government should be able to provide money for an expanding system of herbal education by building herbal schools, and providing botanical gardens, where all sorts of herbs would be planted. The popular demand or the aspiration of the herbalists has been confined to the building of indigenous hospital and herbal college. It is then, they claim that the benefit of herbal drugs could be realised and thus provide adequate health services to the people.

In these distressing days, the use of simple natural drugs would prevent much suffering and save money. The most important subject for people to study, should be: How can we live our allotted time without suffering? God has surely made this possible. *Revolutionise the common manner of living, eating and drinking and you will have a happier and healthier people.*

The Heavenly Father said in Hosea, Ch. 4 Verse 6, that my people were destroyed for lack of knowledge. A lack of knowledge based on truth is accountable for much of the untold sufferings and miseries of humanity.

Education in African society should aim at evolving a true African personality. Such a personality should assimilate for its growth the best in Western and other Civilisations without losing the autonomy of its personality. African cultures should not be allowed to be eroded by the Western civilisation. It is clear that a cultural revolution is now on in Africa, for, African cultures had been largely affected by Western cultures as a result of the continent's historical past. This was unfortunate, because instead of upholding the tradition of their fathers, they have allowed it to waste away in return for the Western cultures as brought by the colonial masters. In order to halt this trend and to succeed with the process of rediscovery which had already begun, they should have confidence in themselves and develop the ability to instill the essence of cultural and ethnic identity. This should be in all fields, such as cultures, art, health services and even in literary and physical education. This is necessary for the growth and expansion of their cultural heritage.

HOW I ACQUIRED THE KNOWLEDGE OF
TRADITIONAL MEDICINE

J. O. Mume, Ph.D.

I had my early training in traditional medicine far back when I was ten. My grandmother's cousin who was a great master of traditional medicine taught me many things to prepare me as healer, a healer of the sick by the African native system of medicine. I was taught healing methods such as massage, bloodletting, herbalism or herbal medicine, hydro-therapy and oracle-telling which I later dropped because of my religious belief and inclination. I was always given the opportunity to sit close to my master, who in the course of training had allowed me to watch the oracle and to read out the meaning to our patients, and my interpretations used to receive the approval of my teacher and as well worked well with the patients.

In herbal medicine I was taught names of more than nine hundred different plants and their medicinal usage. I had the duty of going to the far kokodo forests to gather these plants to see that our pharmacy section was not deficient in valuable medicines. I had to go often to the forest to collect fresh herbs in small quantities, because we had no proper means of preserving them. The only means that was known to us was to burn some of the plants into black powder and store it in dry clay pots and keep them above the fireplace. If we felt that the curative properties of a plant would be destroyed through this process, then we would bury it beneath the earth to be exhumed when the need for its use had arrived.

Going to the bush to collect herbs was most interesting work. It afforded me an opportunity to have time to make use of my catapult to shoot with stones the wild birds, some of whose feathers we use for medicines and the flesh we used for Amiedi soup. I ate a lot of cock meat when I was with my master. These were given to us by our patients as gifts, and our meat container was not at any time found empty, for every serious patient must come to us with at least one fowl. We told them we use the cocks for sacrifice to the dead and the gods, but we eat them in secret. I cannot remember how much we ate under this pretence, but I knew master was not telling the truth to our patients about what happened to the bodies of the cocks. They went into our stomachs when we told them they were meant for the gods and dead.

My master did not believe that the fowls brought by the patients contain some curative elements, but his first demand from patients was always for a cock. We realised that the cure comes from the herbs and roots which our patients took, and cock demand was mere professional tactics and formalities of enriching the doctor's meat-pot. The fowls' legs and necks were for me as meat, and I ate several cock legs in the traditional concept that an apprentice native doctor or follower of a native doctor is the one that eats such organs. But in my modern practice of traditional medicine, I do not demand cocks from my patients. What I demand nowadays is a consultation fee that will be sufficient for me to purchase a cock from the market.

In my advanced training in traditional medicine, I was taught anatomy and surgery. Children's dead bodies, including adults', were cut open to find out the cause of death and to learn the names of internal organs. The study was so excessive that I was taught to know all the names of human organs in my native tongue and tell of their functions. For instance the gall bladder, called "ukpaphe" in Yoruba, is an organ of anger. And people whose bile ducts are misfunctioning have been reported to behave aggressively and irrationally.

We used special native knives in dissecting the bowels of dead patients to see what killed them. We would want to know whether our patients were killed by poisons they were secretly given to eat by witches or wizards, and then to consult the oracle to find out the evildoer.

I had a lot of training in massage and bonesetting. Broken bones of accident victims were mended together with this method and herbal medication.

At the end of my training, my master called me into one deep room and asked me to sit to receive my final instructions in traditional medicine. He told me that the time had come to equip me with the power of clairvoyance—the power which would enable me to see strange things which are quite invisible to others. He went on further, saying that he would put me on his back the following day (Edewor), which is regarded as a special day for that purpose, and on his back we shall both engage in astral travel into the unknown. At this stage I became so terribly frightened. I had earlier been told by our ancestors that only the witches and wizards can fly in the air and travel to their meeting places. So I could not help controlling myself to ask my master, "Are you a wizard?" He nodded his head and gave me an answer which was quite irrlevant to my question.

I hated to become a wizard. Wizardry was not in my blood. My mother was killed by a witch. I knew not of what killed my father, I was too young at the time. Wizards are wicked beings whose inclinations are bent on doing evil against their neighbours all the time. I did not want to specialise in doing evil, but in healing the sick. I made this clear to my teacher who at once understood by mind, and he talked less about taking me along to wizards' meetings.

He told me he was trying to impart in me a full knowledge of African medicine, and as a boy who was so humble and keen he would not like to give me half and half knowledge. But I was not ready to study to become a wizard. That was very obvious to me.

Our class for that day was over, postponed till the following day. When the day arrived, my instructor invited me again into a private room to prepare me for a special knowledge. He brought a special solution prepared of herbal materials and asked me to open my eyes and he poured the solution into them. For over an hour I was uncomfortable and fell into a state of deep trance. When I woke up from a deep sleep, I found myself generating esoteric powers which gave me increased ability of clairvoyance to identify the witches and wizards of our street. They were so many. On one occasion I saw a witch, through this acquired power, walking on her head instead of legs. I was more terrified when I saw another one walking on head with a large cassava basket carried on her legs. She was a close relative who had been previously confessed by another young wizard. I couldn't resist from asking, so I approached her and asked why she chose to carry a load on her legs instead of her head. With a very high emotional tone she said, "Who told you I am carrying a load on my legs? Ekuyoo!"—meaning "Persecution! Persecution! I am being persecuted, I am being persecuted!" Wizards will not readily agree they are wizards. "So you are a witch," I said. In retaliation she told me I was also a wizard; if not, how did I know she was a witch? I comforted her not to be annoyed. But she had been offended, and I suffered the effect of her annoyance, when in the night I received a severe beating from strange hands, with a voice calling my name and saying, "You follower of Mr. Ilarhe, you have been inspired to identify the witches of this town. We shall continue to visit you like this every night for the next one year, and we shall force you to leave this area and Mr. Ilarhe your master cannot help you."

When I woke, I became so wonderfully terrified and sick at heart, casting blame on my master who had imparted this knowledge of knowing wizards at a glance. Afterwards I was living among them in peace for many years, and they have not hurt me, except that I was told my mother was poisoned to death. I was the first to knock at the door of my master to wake him from sleep to tell him about my experiences in the night. He laughed and laughed and laughed, and after a few minutes relaxation he asked, "Did you tell anybody yesterday that she was walking on her head instead of legs?" To this I answered "Yes." Then he went to a nearby bush and gathered some herbs and roots and put them in water for me to bathe in. He then inflicted deep cuts on my arms and forehead and rubbed some black powder into the cuts, and he assured me that I have been immunised against witch attack.

When the night came, I was completely free from strange molestations and I heard not a single voice of threat. I was specially protected with *Ekpofia* and *Amredje* protective and avoidance preparations. These preparations and traditional inoculations made it possible for wizards of our village to avoid me. Although I was avoided and protected, my social life was affected as I lost so many companions and people whom I regarded as faithful friends but who suddenly turned to hate me for no just cause. Their late attitudes towards me gave me good reasons to be suspicious of them.

I quarreled with nobody. So it became so strange that some people in our town suddenly turned to be my enemies. I was not too surprised at this. The woman I saw walking on her head must have betrayed me.

I still possess a scar on my forehead, which is evidence of the inflicted cut of traditional immunisation treatment. People say the scar fits my face. I don't know how far that is true.

The study of traditional medicine to become a qualified native doctor is an intricate one. One has got to learn curative and destructive methods that are unknown to medical doctors and unbelievable by them. Medical doctors want tests and proof, and when they have proved, they condemn again. Our proofs are the results.

Finally I was invited to the private room again by my master, and after giving me more oral instructions on the accepted rules that will guide me in identification of witches and wizards, he poured another herbal solution, this time not into my eyes but my ears. Although I did not fall into a state of trance, as in the eye-opening experience, my head became heavy, and I felt a crawling movement in my head and I began to feel increased power moving me to hear strange sounds, and to generate a force which was enabling me to understand the linguistic songs of birds and animals. Seven days later when I was sent to gather herbs in the forest, a friendly bird sang a song which I perfectly understood to mean, "Danger is in front, return home, return home." I returned home. And another occasion when a similar song of warning was sung to me by a bird the Yorubas call "Agbrere," I disobeyed his predictive voice and returned home in agony and with wounds I sustained when I fell into a deep fishpond as a result of slippery ground. The squirrel, called "Ota" in Yoruba, is a small bush animal that is skilled in prediction. I had once disobeyed a squirrel's prediction warning me of danger when I was going on my same herbal mission. I returned home temporarily blinded when a cobra sprayed saliva on my eyes.

My master was kind and powerful, but he used to be wicked at times. He taught me kindness and prepared a path which would make me great. He was fond of calling me by my

140

native name "Ojo" with the addition of an adjectival word, "great." Thus the name he was calling me was "Ojo the Great." Dr. Ilarhe was really a wonderful man, and I have reasons for my conviction. One of his powerful aspects is his ability to identify witches, mention people's names on first sight, and tell their past and present life stories. Once he predicted to one famous Tsekri Chief who came to consult him that his senior son would die within twenty-one days. He really died before the period.

I remember in 1942 when my master had a land dispute with another native doctor of repute. Both challenged each other in root power, and I heard my master telling his rival that he would not live to see the seventh day. The same word was repeated to my master by his opponent. Then it was for us, learner doctors, to watch whose power will surpass the other. I saw my master fortifying himself with native preparations against wizard's attack and, as well, sending powerful destructive spells telepathically to his opponent. In the early morning of the third day after their quarrel, there were shouts that Mr. X had died. The Mr. X was the rival of my master. He was struck to death by lightening which penetrated his thick mud wall to strike him while in bed.

The news made my master sad, but never for long. The sadness was turned to joy when master bought an all-white ram which he slaughtered to make a sacrificial dinner party. Few people attended the party because every person had reason to attribute the cause of Mr. X's death to my master. Some openly said Mr. X was killed by Dr. Ilarhe. Otherwise, how could his rival die a few days after they quarreled? "Mr. Ilarhe is wicked, Mr. Ilarhe is powerful," was the current news of the time.

In due course the family of the late opponent came to my master to beg him not to take the life of another member of their family. They brought to my master a he-goat and materials with which to cook it, and the disputed land also was surrendered to him, closing every matter relating to the land dispute.

From that time on, I started to fear my master the more and to submit myself fully in all the messages he sent me. I was tremendously increasing in the power of clairvoyance from day to day, and my street witches who were aware of this fact were cleverly getting rid of me. At this time they had all turned to walk on legs as human beings do. By this they thought they were preventing me from recognising them as witches and wizards. One day to my horror I saw my master Dr. Ilarhe walking on his head, and I became convinced that although he devoted his ability to the healing of the sick, he was also a member of the night club, and holds a title of "Adjele."

I am a highly religious man, but at times there used to be backsliding because of imperfections which we all inherited from our parents. I was made to believe through my acquired powers that the Almighty God will one day destroy the wicked and only righteous beings will remain and live on earth forever. I want to live forever, so I joined the religion which my esoteric power directed, through which I can survive a great battle to live. My religion uses the Bible and I wholeheartedly believe in it.

Then came my graduation day. Everything was prepared for the occasion. Many people were invited, including noted native doctors, witch doctors, bonesetters, herbalists, to see me receive my white cap which qualified me to be initiated to the Urhobo Idiebo Society. From that time on I became the "Obo," meaning healer or doctor. This happened in 1944, and after serving my master for another year, I was finally left on my own, but I did not open up practice. I wanted to be educated, and to devote more time to the study of my Bible and the practice of my religion. Because of certain conflicts between my clairvoyance and the Bible doctrines, I surrendered myself in favour of the Bible. The Bible teaches that we should have more friends. But I have lost so many good friends and made more enemies for being clairvoyant. And today I have no more desire to indulge in the esoteric exercise of witch revelation. It is a practice that is more risky, and the sort that tends to retard social and economic progress.

Not every person that confesses to witchcraft is really a witch. There are some people who impersonate witches and wizards who know nothing about witchery and how to walk on the head. They are falsely parading themselves as such to make people fear them and look upon them as gods. Some are also pretending to be so in order to dupe patients to give them money. Such impostors have suffered in the hands of true wizards, some were even killed through supernatural means. A true wizard will not at all confess he is, unless under the pressure of a lingering disease and when he fully realises that he will surely die. Some wizards used to take delight in confessing their wicked deeds when they were about to pass away. This is because they know that the dead know nothing.

Although I was guided halfway by my master on the path to become a wizard, never had I wished to be established as a wizard. I had only thought of becoming a healer, for there is a great demarcation between witchery and healing. So I decided to be a successful healer—the line to which my religion and ego directed me. Witchery and healing have opposing functions and practices which cannot be coordinated. One stands to destroy, the other stands to prevent and cure.

I decided on the path to prevent and cure diseases in the African native way, and so had to equip myself in the knowledge of treating wizard-infested diseases in the proved traditional way with protective preparations called in Yoruba *Ifue, Ekpofia, Amrevweadje, Akuebe* and *Ariakpa*. These are proved traditional remedies which medical scientists cannot probe into, yet they are effective.

I saw thousands of patients treated by my master Dr. Ilarhe. Among the several kinds of diseases he cured with native methods can be mentioned asthma, colitis, constipation, dropsy, eye troubles, ear troubles, epilepsy, migraine, headaches, menopause, sterility in male and female, insanity, neuroses, stomach troubles, wizard-infested disorders, gonorrhoea, liver disorders and a host of other diseases.

Most of the patients who came to our healing home were patients who had attended the general hospitals, and they all expressed dissatisfaction over the treatment given them. We were able to solve their problems for them by the traditional methods. Some of the patients who were demon-possessed were being haunted day and night and were in constant fear. We used the avoidance preparation called *Amregdje* on such unfortunate patients to case out the demons. This is something the medical doctor cannot do, and also cannot believe.

My master died some years ago, and his practice has been passed unto me and one of his sons, "John Boy Ilarhe," now practicing native medicine at Ekrokpe. My master lived 120 years before he passed away quietly on his bed. Before he died, he predicted the exact date of his death. But he remained on the bed for seven days before he finally stopped to breathe, when other parts of his body had started to rot away. This was because there were some native lifepostponement preparations called "Oberuyovwi" that had to be brought down to stop the last breath. Having done this, he died completely and he was given a decent burial.

Before he died, he confessed his sins before the world, and told his people that, although he was a great healer, he was also a killer; for he took the lives of seven people to qualify for the title of "Adjele" in the witchery club. And that is why in his later years he had to suffer from blindness in order to account for his sins. When he was about to die he called me and gave me his last admonition and reminded me that I have courageously acted wisely to have refused membership in the night club; otherwise I would have suffered in the same manner of his last days. This I well realised, and the religion which I embraced had taught me more about the wages of sin and about a particular law of the Bible which says, "Thou shalt not kill."

When he was fast breathing to leave this world, he placed his right hand on my head and called me in a deteriorated voice, "Ojo the Great, Ojo the Great. You are really going to be great, and your name will become a household name in Nigeria and in all the world. The rulers shall all come to know you through the work of native medicine [Ebo], and you shall be a pioneer in the field of traditional medicine, and other native doctors shall come to learn at your feet. I know your way will be hard at first, but you will succeed in spite of the opposition and the jealousy of western-trained doctors."

He asked me to bring a native white chalk (Oren) and when I brought it, he broke it and put some quantity into my right hand and rubbed some on my forehead and said: "Let everything I have showed unto you be effective to your patients [*osekewe*]." To this I answered, "Ise," meaning "Amen." After this he breathed his last breath and passed away from this world, passing his knowledge into my hands.

Many medical doctors and health workers have condemned practitioners of the native system because they have been blinded by their own faith and would not want to see other points of view. Very few have studied our beliefs for even a few days, and have then felt competent to know all about the subject of traditional medicine and to interpret and make known that which takes our cleverest doctor of native medicine a lifetime to discover. Medical doctors cannot honestly guide the policy of traditional medicine because they are not trained in it.

People who criticize traditional medicine are those whose acceptance-rejection phenomenon is conditioned by the magic of foreign names and colonial mentality and an unquestionable acceptance of the myth that nothing good can ever come out of Africa. It is a candid truth that their assertions are not based on any empirical data or experience whatsoever but strictly on sentiments, jealousy and hatred for anything bearing the label of "native" or "tradition." There is nothing short of the truth that the medical doctors could learn so much from traditional doctors, if the medical doctors were not arrogant and would be willing to cooperate. Several medical doctors who have witnessed the results of my treatments and were not proud to refuse to attend some of my lectures on traditional medicine have expressed deep interest in traditional medicine, but invariably they say that I should carry on my activities and propagation of traditional medicine until the government would do something, but that I should not mention their names as that would prejudice their reputation. What a nonsense!

After my education in various primary schools in my area, I proceeded to Lagos in 1945 in pursuit of further education, but broke up my studies at Eko Boys High School for lack of financial support. After much hardship in Lagos, I returned home in 1950 with my heart fixed on establishing a herbal clinic at my hometown Ekakpamre in a modernized form. On the basis of the practical knowledge I had gained from my grandmother's cousin, I set up a herbal clinic where I was curing the sick as well as conducting more research and probing into the secret treasure of Yoruba traditional medicine, and later covering the whole Federation of Nigeria. The adventure took me to many places such as Okitipupa, Ilesha, Ife, Oshogbo, Idanre, Enugu, Owerri, Calabar, Yola, Benin City, contacting prominent native doctors and herbalists, gaining experience and valuable therapeutic knowledge.

I was practicing in a little room which I inherited from my father until I started to think of building a separate house purposely for the clinic. Although there are very many old houses in our compound where I could have practiced, I felt there was need for a house to portray the traditional outlook befitting the kind of work I have determined to do for life. It is significant to note that the first house I built for the practice was built at that time for a cost of two pounds ten shillings. You can imagine what such a house would look like. It was a small mud-walled and thatch-roofed house apportioned into two rooms. After two years it appeared success was trying to laugh at me, and so I built another house, this time at a cost of ten pounds. They were little houses built in the pattern of my old master.

But I did not stop at that. I realised that before one can really succeed in any undertaking, he must first acquire knowledge, and knowledge comes from learning. I also realised that whatever the mind of man can conceive and believe it can achieve.

My next task, therefore, was to conduct further and further research into the tropical medicinal plants in the way they were used by our fathers, the native doctors and herbalists, in order to modernise the traditional system of cure. The exercise cost me several pounds in cash and nuts of kola. Most of the native doctors and herbalists I met were pecuniary-minded and very uncompromising in revealing their therapeutic methods. In spite of this difficulty and uncompromising attitude, I was still able to win the hearts of some experienced and kind practitioners through open hands of financial gifts, and the task required much skill.

While doing all this I was also intricately mindful of

how I will improve my standard of general education. I became much involved in planning for the future, and the thought was always with me that the college or university classroom is not necessarily the only place meant for the acquisition of education. Education does not consist of sitting idly with one's head and arms resting on the college bench. It is acquired by studying books, by experience in doing, by imitation, by travel and meeting people and by positive development of mind. I was so faithfully guided by my ego to believe that I could improve my educational standard up to the grade of Ph.D. through private studies. This is a dream which I have already realised in my home through study in selected books and by correspondence tuition.

At the initial end of such strenuous research, I came to have my own modified materia medica of forty herbal medicines which include traditional immunisation preparations which can protect one from the attacks of witches and wizards of the kinds I had from my master, and which I have been using in my clinic since then. During this time, my work became known throughout the Yoruba tribe and all parts of Nigeria. I became known as the first educated Nigerian that ranged the woods and climbed the hills in search of medicinal herbs for the service of humanity. During much of that time I engaged in research and healing work directed to the seemingly incurable diseases and to prevent and cure such diseases that are caused by wicked hands of witches and wizards. I was so richly blessed with success that in spite of the fact that I was working twice as many hours as does the so-called "working man," I was exceedingly happy.

But never, at any time, did I resort to the use of English medicines or drugs to mix up with the traditional remedies which I use. To have done so would have been hypocritical and ridiculous. Although there were so many herbalists who claim to practice in the traditional way, it did not take me much time to know that they were abusing and misusing their gift of healing by mixing up with foreign drugs and some were even administering illegal injections to their patients. The pertinent thing to note in this is that such practices are a corruption of traditional medicine, and a deviation from the true philosophy of traditional healing.

In 1955 when I had practiced for five years, news came to me that some American Naturopathic physicians had arrived in Nigeria to set up a school of Natural Therapeutics, whose aims were to teach all branches of natural healing, including herbal medicine, massage, biochemic therapy, naturopathy, osteopathy, and zone therapy. My interest was aroused, so I applied as a part-time student and paid my fees from the money I earned as a news vendor. The school's address was 9 Abulenla Road, Ebute-Metta, Lagos. I enrolled at the school to study herbalism, biochemic therapy and naturopathy. But the school did not stay long in Nigeria, for reasons not fully disclosed to us by the American principal when he was asked to leave. But the reason was not too difficult for us to understand. From time to time in all parts of the world, practitioners of traditional medicine and nature cure have been persecuted by members of the medical profession, and in spite of this medical monopoly, the traditional methods of healing continue to become more and more popular among the simple and intellectual classes.

Afterwards, I returned home to Ekakpamre and started afresh, and with the knowledge I gained from the school at Lagos, I started to plan, to meditate, to read, to develop and improve upon my traditional herbal products which I prepared in powder and liquid. My whole object in this successful research was to find and correct these derangements, so as to place my patients in a better state of natural resistance to disease. My whole idea was to acquire such deep and hiding knowledge of traditional medicine as would enable me to do for my patients what would give natural healing the best possible chance to succeed.

In fact, it was because of this achievement that I became known as a practitioner of traditional medicine among many people all over Nigeria and some other parts of the world. "Seek and ye shall find" is a promise which is being wonderfully fulfilled in connection with traditional medicine, and I have always been motivated to think that, if our forefathers could treat and cure the various diseases which afflict human beings with native herbs and other simple natural methods, why can such methods not be investigated and developed in a better way by us? This is a question I frequently ask myself, and to get an answer has kept me busy in constant research to this day.

What is worth doing is worth doing well. And so with the address of Oversea Colleges I got from our leaving principal at Lagos, I started taking a series of correspondence courses in naturopathy, herbalism, biochemic therapy and osteopathy.

During the period, I was combining too many duties together: visiting the virgin forests to collect herbs, roots, bark and seeds; and preparing them for commercial taste; taking them to the consumers in our vehicle, sometimes alone and sometimes with my other partners. The pressure of duty became too heavy on me and in 1957 when our partnership broke down and our van had been sold for £35 at the loss of £300, I too broke down in health, not necessarily because of business failure but perhaps because I had over-laboured myself when I had no time to relax, and what I was eating then was imbalanced food richer in carbohydrates, I came to understand.

In 1956 I moved my practice to Orho-Agbarho, my maternal place of birth, where I now live. Here at Agbarho it did not take much time before people began to notice my activities. Within six months, my own success in cases where orthodox treatment had been of no avail was so great and so frequent that a great deal of my time was taken up with explaining to so many enquirers how the cures were brought about. I used to explain to these people how the traditional system of medicine had provided what these very sick people desperately needed in order not to die, and also why particular preparations were enabling them to regain good health.

Soon there were quite a number of prominent people of all walks of life who had first-hand knowledge of how my patients were rescued from death or chronic invalidism. I began to be consulted by some of them. Even some who claim to be practitioners of orthodox medicine have consulted me in secret and have witnessed results of the treatment—which, it is not too much to say, have astonished them.

During all this time, the Nigerian press was aware of my activities but refused to publish them. It seems perhaps they were watching to see more of my progress, and so I was surprised when one day while engaged in my work, my receptionist informed me that I had press visitors from Benin whose intentions were to interview me about the work I am doing. I invited them in and formal introduction revealed them as N.M. Ukoli, editor of the *Sunday Observer*, Mike Ajari, sub-editor, and their photographer. The interview was published in the *Sunday Observer* of November 24, 1968, and I was termed in the headline as the "man who can cure all diseases with traditional medicine."

I was thrilled to see myself and my work in print for the first time, and at once realised that I am doing a worthwhile work and began immediately to set my hands on harder work, replying to enlighten more and more people who wanted to know about my clinic and of my healing ability. The press gave me greater confidence in my work.

The time has come to engage in more extensive research work, and at the same time directing the building of my clinic and residence which I completed in 1969 at a total cost of £2,000 and officially opened on February 10. While so engaged, I was also seriously working on a thesis for the doctor of philosophy degree in Naturopathy, a more technical term for natural methods of treating diseases which can be regarded in Nigeria as traditional medicine. On May 11, 1970, I submitted a thesis covering the subject, "Natural Dietetics, Traditional Medicine in Nigeria and Biochemic-Therapy" to the International University of Kanpur, India, through the college of Natural Therapeutics, Diyatalawa, Ceylon. I was overwhelmed with joy to hear that I passed the degree with distinction, and today I am a holder of a Ph.D. in Naturopathy, in other words a doctorate in traditional medicine.

I happen to be the first man to hold this qualification in Nigeria (I am not sure of the whole of Africa). When the news of my success broke out through all the news media of Nigeria, it became a pressing thing for people of all ranks including Nigerian higher institutions, universities, herbalists associations, colleges and cultural societies to invite me to deliver lectures on my special field of activities, and possibly to put my work into writing. In submission to such requests from well-meaning friends, I have written a book on traditional medicine in Nigeria, now in the hands of the publishers, and I hope the book will serve as an introduction to the philosophy and principle of Nigerian traditional medicine and a source of information on African healing science. I hope you will be delighted to understand that the foreword to the book was written by Professor A. Akisanya of the chemistry department of Lagos University, who is a respected scholar who has devoted part of his time probing the chemical constituents of African herbal medicines.

Today it is common knowledge that some of the most serious ailments to which the human race is prone can be successfully treated by the traditional natural methods where orthodox medicine has failed.

While medical doctors are working to suppress the activities of traditional doctors and always speaking in terms of ridicule against traditional medicine, my fight has always been for the revival and development of traditional medicine, and I have always maintained my peace with my aggressors and those regarding me as a medical impostor. I have always made them realise that traditional medicine is a transmitted culture of the people which treats diseases of the body and mind, as well as culture-bound diseases.

Having now come to realise the cultural importance of traditional healing methods, it becomes absolutely necessary to formulate a sound policy for the revival and development of traditional medicine. The traditional methods of healing disease cannot be blown away by the winds, because their roots reach deep into the soil. Traditional medicine has its own philosophies and bears a separate identity, and so we cannot allow orthodox medicine to virtually absorb our methods of healing. Any attempt by any person or group of persons to pervert and annihilate the basic principle and practice of our fathers' healing act will be vehemently and supernaturally resisted by the native doctors and herbalists.

In the rest of this paper, I would like to discuss some aspects of traditional psychiatry and present two case histories. In Nigeria, the traditional psychiatric treatment of mental cases consisted in torturing the patient in order to drive out of him the devil and evil spirits to whom the suffering was attributed. Various forms of torture were known, but the most regarded is the beating with medicated broom or stick. This method may be regarded in some quarters as brutal treatment, but to the traditional physician it is not as brutal as the drug and electrical convulsive treatment generally administered in mental hospitals, with their corresponding side effects.

I will not entirely condemn electrical convulsive treatment. E.C.T. is acceptable to me not on the claims attached to it by the inventor, but on my very personal belief that E.C.T. application can disturb or disorganise the peaceful existence of evil spirits in demon-possessed patients.

Apart from beating such patients to drive away the evil spirits, the traditional psychiatrist is of the opinion that when violence is applied to violence the resultant end is peace and harmony. This means, when a violent mental patient is treated with some form of therapeutic violence, the patient's healing force is stimulated to produce a curative reaction which makes him calm and less violent. At this stage of cheerfulness, the traditional psychiatrist will then have a suitable time to investigate the cause or causes of his patient's abnormal behaviour. He asks psychological investigative questions to determine whether his patient had committed some evil deeds, and if this is confirmed, then the only means of cure is to persuade the patient to confess his sins and let him be forgiven through prayers and sacrifices by the family elders with the traditional psychiatrist directing the whole affair.

In some cases when mental disorders are due to anxieties as a result of business failures, or loss of a dear one through death and improperly planned love affairs, the traditional physician would give all necessary advice and encouragements that will enable his patient to recover quickly from his depressive state and start to live a useful life again. This is what the medical psychiatrist will not do, and this is a very good reason why mental cases have defeated them. Shock treatment cannot solve the patient's internal conflicts, it will only send the patient into a state of coma temporarily and he awakes to be confronted again with the same thoughts of guilt which had brought his mental problems, which only prayers of forgiveness can remove.

Another factor responsible for mental disorders as seen by the traditional doctors is "chemical imbalance" or deficiency of essential elements. That is, if the brain is deprived of certain chemical elements such as phosphates, potassium, etc., through unbalanced dieting and the like, then mental disorder can develop. The only sensible way is to correct the dietetic error and fortify the body with the needed materials by means of good food and herbal remedies.

Another very important cause of brain trouble is subluxation or displacement of the vertebrae of the spine. This can cause pressure on the nerves passing through that section, and thus cause disorders in the organs controlled by the nerves of that section of the nerves passing through the spinal cord. The treatment generally adopted by traditional practitioners in this case is by methodical manipulation and gentle pressure on the spine or concussion, i.e., a blow with the hand on the subluxated section to bring about healing of the disorder of those organs.

Many practitioners of traditional medicine practice these forms of psychosomatic therapeutics intuitively because most of them treat patients who come from the organically-minded doctors who have told these patients that they can do no more to help their functional disorders. The Nigerian native doctors have accomplished much and pioneered in mental therapy and other forms of healing.

As I said earlier, I am not attempting to teach psychiatry but only trying to acquaint my audience with the facts that the traditional methods of treating mental disorders are quite different to that practiced by the medical psychiatrists, and the traditional methods are quite safer and effective.

I would like to relate two case histories of my psychiatric patients whom I successfully treated.

Case No. 1

Mr. K., age thirty-two years, told me he had consulted

quite a number of doctors and had taken all kinds of drugs and received shock treatment in one of the country's oldest mental hospitals, until he was wholly disgusted with it all. He said his troubles were growing worse and the thought of committing suicide was always by him.

When I enquired further, he told me he was being chased day and night by the dead ancestors who wanted to kill him. My investigation revealed that the patient was not suffering from any organic disorder but his case was purely a functional one, which requires suggestive treatment.

I probed deep in the traditional method of diagnosing such cases. He confessed through my persuasion that he had committed a sin by having sexual intercourse with the father's junior wife, and this now was generating inner conflict in him which led to his brain trouble. He feared to see the father. The slightest sight of his father would make him run amok and cry aloud that he was being haunted by the dead. He said he would give all he had if he could be cured.

I told him I could help him if he would cooperate. He agreed to do as directed. I knew the way to cure him. It was not a case for tablets or beating. I accompanied him to see his people and asked him to openly confess his sins before his family so that he would be forgiven. He did so, and with much pressure I persuaded the father and the elders to offer sincere prayers of forgiveness in the customary way. After a very long pleading to calm their unpleasant emotions, they agreed to do what I asked. The family's spokesman requested my patient to buy a goat, yams and plantain, seven big cola-nuts and the rest of it. My patient had financially exhausted himself and had no means of providing these items. I knew that this was the only means by which I could cure my patient. So out of my meager resources I bought the goat and all the other materials and went with my patient to meet his family after seven days' time. The family elders were all present, the goat was killed and cooked, and prayers of forgiveness were offered by the most elder who pronounced that my patient's troubles were now over, but that he should not commit such grievous sin again. His guilty conscience was released, and he started to develop confidence and cheerfulness. Within ten days his sanity returned. I prescribed Akata

154

root in powder to strengthen his nerves, and I also instructed him to eat only natural foods and forget about his past mistakes. He thanked me and declared that no medical psychiatrist would have succeeded in solving his trouble, as none would have been able to understand the root cause of his ailment and approach his family for such a cooperative treatment.

I discharged him in three weeks, and I saw him two years later with a happy expression in his face and feeling pretty good. He has since taken an appointment with a company as assistant secretary.

Is anyone sick among you? Let him call for the elders of the church (family); and let them pray over him, anointing him with oil in the name of the Lord. And the prayer of faith shall save the sick, and the Lord shall raise him up; and if he have committed sins, they shall be forgiven him. Confess your faults one to another, and pray one for another, that ye may be healed. The effectual fervent prayer of a righteous man availeth much (James 5.14-16).

Case No. 2

Mrs. N.E., twenty-seven years old, gave birth to a male child and went mad. Her illness immediately after delivery was malaria fever, frequent colds, and headache. Symptomatically she has dizziness, high temperature, sleeplessness, fetid breath, great fear and strong desire to move about.

When she started to give me details of her illness, she could not raise her face to look at me, and was very reluctant to talk. The only thing she could say was, "I have a mighty snake going up and down in my stomach trying to take my life." She wept and said she would die the following day through the aggressive behaviour of the snake that was going up and down in her bowel.

She stood up and shouted, "Doctor, can you remove this snake from my belly? I have been to so many medical psychiatrists who could not help me." Hers was a real case of insanity.

I assured her in the presence of her husband, who looked

so desperate, that I would cure her trouble. She asked whether I could kill the big snake in her body. I told her this is something traditional medicine can do, and I requested that she should remain with me for my personal supervision.

After half of my bill had been settled, I gave her Akata root powder, a herbal sedative which sent her to a deep sleep. She felt better with the first dose, although she complained of the same snake. I assured her that in seven days I would kill the snake in her bowel, and she would see it. She laughed and said that there was no one that could kill the snake, unless God. I told her that I am an ambassador blessed by God to heal the afflicted ones.

When the seventh day arrived, I sent my assistants, whom I had previously immunised against snake bite poison, to the bush to bring a big snake back, dead or alive. One of my assistants succeeded in bringing one dead. I kept it in a bottle, taking care my patient did not see it.

When everything was ready, I called my patient and gave her a herbal emetic to cause vomiting. When she started to vomit, I rubbed pepper into her eyes in order to blackmail her from knowing my therapeutic tricks. While she closed her eyes as a result of the pepper application, and at the same time vomiting as a result of the medicine I gave her, I secretly removed the big snake from the bottle and placed it among her vomit and asked her to open her eyes; only to see a dead snake in front of her. I shouted in an unusual voice, "Your trouble is now over, your trouble is now over. I have killed the snake that is going up and down in your stomach, and I have made you to vomit it. Your trouble is over." Her trouble and all the associated symptoms disappeared in a few minutes.

Her face filled with joy as she expressed her gratitude to me that her trouble was really over. She asked me to keep the snake for her husband to see to confirm all that she had been saying about a wicked snake in her bowel. When her husband came to see her, she was the first person to bring the snake to his attention, and said, "This is what I have been telling you that there was a snake in my stomach and you people would say I was mad. Now my madness has been cured by the ambassador of God."

The husband asked me whether it was a fact his wife had actually vomited a snake. I was not prepared to speak the truth. That remains a professional secret to me. "Look at your wife, is she not now cured? What else do you want?"

Do you call me a trickster? I agree, but I have done my job. I discharged her after my balance had been paid, and gave her a sufficient quantity of herbal preparations to be taken at home. It is over ten years, and the lady is still going about in all life activities and has no feeling of snake movement in her abdomen.

Traditional medicine stands on its own entity, and its methods and principles of treating diseases are quite practical and natural, and different from the orthodox medical system. That is why the orthodox medical practitioners cannot honestly direct the policy of traditional medicine.

I hope the time will soon come when the Federal Military Government will overcome all pressures by the western trained doctors and advisers, to embark on a gigantic plan to revive and develop the traditional medical system for the benefit of humanity.

THE DUALITY OF TRADITIONAL AND WESTERN MEDICINE IN AFRICA: MYSTICS, MYTHS AND REALITY*

F. M. Mburu, Ph.D.

I. Introduction

The research on which the present paper is based was conducted from April, 1972, to April, 1974, among the Akamba ethnic group of Machakos District, Kenya. The data used in this paper was obtained through participant observation when the author lived among the people.

During the research period the author compared his work with the work of a visiting non-African sociologist interested in the same area of study. It became evident that the non-African was more acceptable to the traditional herbalists and diviners than the African was. The acceptance of the latter by the lay population was overwhelming in comparison. The rejection of an African student by his kith and kin is a phenomenon reported by others in various fields of investigations like journalism, where African leaders would rather give interviews to foreign journalists than to indigenous reporters. In very many respects, the African traditional doctor is more at home with foreigners because he, erroneously considers them ignorant of his modus operandi and modus vivendi. The White person is a temporary visitor without any interests, and even if he had any at all, what does he know about "our customs?" The fellow native is a threat to the traditional practitioners. He knows too much, is likely to let out secrets, he might be spying for a rival practitioner and, if educated, ipso facto, he must be a government agent, brain-washed by colonial epithets and obviously someone to keep at arms' length. Modern education is a paradoxical achievement; at once an asset desired by many, at once a stigma in rationalizing some outrageously obnoxious African inferiority complex.

---

*I am indebted to Dr. Mickey C. Smith and Dr. John Furr for the benefit of their comments on a draft of this paper.

Often, however, this degree of rejection is not without some grain of justification. If African traditional medicine has been chastised, the native elite has done it most. The White man has been more open where the African, particularly the modern physician, violently shuts out any interchange of ideas with the traditional specialist. In the three East African medical schools the African future physician at best does not want to hear anything about the traditional healing system, at worst he is enthusiastically hostile to patients who confess patronizing traditional medicine, less expensive as it is. There is, therefore, mutual hostility. The lack of perceived mutual benefit and the omnipresent idiosyncratic cynicism vis-a-vis the other system makes it extremely hard to gouge a common goal.

The present paper describes the relevance of both the traditional and modern medicine to an indigenous population. It explores the conflicts resultant from the interaction of discordant belief systems, interest groups, fear of dismemberment and sheer ignorance of the dynamics of the alien system vis-a-vis the indigenous. The relationship between the modern physician and the traditional specialist is compounded by a colonial history. A hard and fast prescription on how to handle the relationship would hardly stand the test of time and would not be a sensible frame of reference. Personality types, political expediencies, socioeconomic interests cannot be too comfortably ignored. But no prognostications are made here. The first person singular is used to avoid any unwarranted theoretical pretentions and the intellectual potholes therein.

II. African Cosmology in Contemporary Medical Practice

Human societies are full of contradictions in every realm of life. People who consider themselves modernized often harbor some traits of their experiential past in their behavior though they are not conscious that they carry such left-overs in their every day life. Such traits, unless in diametric opposition to modern ideas, are considered modern by way of rationalization. For instance, in the realm of

African politics are some of the greatest radicals in the continent. They clamor for dramatic changes according to individual ideological inclination. They preach political nationalization as opposed to provincial and parochial tribal groupings. Yet, almost to a man, some of the artifacts displayed by these political elites to legitimize their authority have traditional underpinnings, very often of the leader's ethnic group. The late Kwame Nkrumah was at once a Western-type philosopher and a tribal Osagyefo or the "redeemer." The latter was more of a kingly title for 'a person deeply committed to a parliamentary democracy. Today President Nyerere of Tanzania uses African traditional organization to explain and justify socialism.

Such cases in the realm of health are many. They legitimize the past in the present of a person who has here and now wants and needs. During a family planning lecture in a rural area in Kenya, a 47 year old man challenged me in the following way:

> I have two wives and twelve children. We need to reproduce as much as our ancestors did and as fast as we could. Our reproduction is counter-balanced by those of you young men who do neither marry nor work and when they marry they bear no children. Where would you young men get wives if we have no children, anyway? Two, ten, twenty children no difference to anybody; God will provide. Some will go to school, others will be laborers. We bear doctors and thieves.[1]

The argument of this man is sound enough if viewed from conditions pertaining to the lifestyle of former generations long gone by and regardless of the conditions existing now as well as the cost of living this man has to live with. To argue that "some will go to school..." is to be ignorant of the fact that the training of a physician costs much more than the training of a herds boy. The man's implicit assumption is that some children will inevitably die. He seems to believe, as many of us do, that to frequent the hospital is one thing, quite another to fully confide in the efficacy of modern hospital. This belief is exemplified by the following case not far from Nairobi city:

> A mother of six sat outside her hut chatting with four of her children. Another child aged three years and four

months was said to be in bed slightly ill. In fact, when the child was brought to us after a lot of persuasion, we found it to be half dead. The arm circumference was 7.2 cm (3.00"), weighted 5.8 kg. (12.76 lb.) and was a severe case of kwashiorkor. The mother was not in the least in a hurry to take the child to the hospital, probably with good reason.

Another of her daughters aged 14 years, suffered from an advanced stage of lymphodenopathy. She had had it for more than five years. The girl had many times been treated in the national hospital. She was every time withdrawn from the hospital a month or so to continue therapy with well known herbalists. This was on the knowledgeable advice of the neighbors and the relatives. She summed her plight thus:

"since these children are so bad, there is no hope of ever obtaining better medicine than they are getting now. I have given up hospital medicine. They will now follow our Kikamba medicine." When we referred her to the clinic nearby, she tore the referral sheet into pieces in our presence.[2]

To give oneself up to the concept of modern medicine in a community that has had a radically different system of medical concepts is no mean achievement. Illness ideas are very much a function of the social condition of the people, their values, philosophy, attitudes and the conviction that such diseases can or cannot be treated or cured. Among some African tribes a person suffering from, say TB, may be clinically curable, but will neither admit that he has the disease nor seek "competent" medical help. The Kikuyu, Embu, Meru, Kamba, Masai, to name a few, often maintain their preferred health status by just doing nothing about it. Doing something about health is speculating on the capabilities of the Almighty and his anger might be the most probable consequence. Preventive medicine is anathema. How, they ask, can you prevent that which you neither have nor know.[4] The cosmology of these people is based on some very strong and dogmatic religions and myths. Their God is as benevolent as he is ruthless on provocation. To admit illness is ipso facto to admit an error of commission or omission, the last thing many want to do. Medicine and prayers are for the needy, the needless should not pester God with incessant aimless demands. Such people are like those sick who have "nothing wrong" but who should be the focus of all physicians.[5] The uncertainty of health and disease in traditional societies has come a long way from the ancestors. Traditional medicine evaluation is partly based on the beliefs of the society, partly on the value systems, and partly on the actual behavior of the needy client. But modern medicine falls short of this. It is something the people do not understand. It is as foreign as the white faces, coats and buildings associated with it. They are, therefore, asked to have faith in something alien to them; faith has failed them in the past. The little faith there might be is forgotten when faith and scientific reasoning are confused and fail to concur, as often happens. It is a matter of "yes, I know this, but. . . ." Like a man who told me:

> I have had twenty-six children, now I have only six alive. Can you tell me what happened to the other twenty? Why are they not with me? By the time you are half my age you will have stopped talking this family limitation language. I have seen the world, you haven't.[6]

The story this man is telling is that there are two worlds and two systems: the modern for the knowledgeable youth and their pretentious understanding of the world, and the other based on experience of the past. In the past death has been the order, rather than the exception. Children perished in spite of the availability of traditional and modern medicine. They failed to prevail in the time of need. They certainly will fail again.

The science of modern medicine is not being introduced in Africa in a vacuum.[7] These people have had their own system of health maintenance.[8] And they have enough problems with it without having to bother with new things never seen or tested before. The new, therefore, has to impinge on the old, if not to oust it altogether. The new will be effective only when people realize or believe that the quality of care provided is good enough for them but not when some empty prognostications are forced down their throats. In an attempt to show how naively traditional medicine is conceived by what he called "new Africans," a man said:

I was in school when I was struck down by a mysterious coughing spout. My brother took me to Machakos hospital where I was admitted for two weeks without any sign of improvement. Then my father took me home to rest, he said. When I was there he consulted a Mkamba diviner about my condition and was told that some body cast a spell on me. The diviner prescribed that we pay him a goat to undo the evil spell and to protect the whole family from such people. You know we Africans. If cure is not quick, regardless of the type of medicine, we think somebody has used sorcery or witchcraft against us so that illness can go on for eternity. But the African doctor is able to see this and able to determine what makes illness continue. Our diviners see things hospital doctors cannot perceive. Nonetheless, you have to tell the diviner your trouble or else he can't help you. Since my treatment by the traditional doctor, I have been perfect.[9]

The cases above show common mistrust of modern medicine. In these cases we find that the clients first turned to modern medicine before switching to traditional medicine. Again in these cases, the relatives and neighbors of the sick expected an immediate resumption of the preferred status of health, or as Dubos[10] says: "a modus vivendi enabling imperfect man to achieve a reward and not too painful existence while they cope with an imperfect world." It is apparent that the problem with modern medicine is not so much that it does not cure. On the contrary, it does, but fails to operate according to the expectations of the sick and of the community. It purports to give a diagnosis which is hidden from the patient. More often than not the secrecy thereof confirms the fear of the patient that he is in a terrible pathological state. He is made to believe that he is so ill that the physiochemical expert with the aid of mechanical instruments cannot assess the extent of the bacteriological conflict. When he can delineate the dimensions of the damage, the expert finds, so the patient believes, that the microbial destruction is so advanced that it should neither be made public nor made known to the person who happens to be the medium of the conflict.

To alienate the modern physician further from the African patient is the concept of etiology. The physician seeks vindication of his germ-theory stand in the very science to which he is committed. The patient and the relatives neither understand this science nor are committed to it. They, therefore, cannot have a quarrel with the physician. The modern and the traditional have little or no common referents about etiological propensities. The patient and the physician do not contradict each other. The African patient seeks to find the reason *why* it all happened to him, not how it happens to all and sundry. The physician tells him *what* usually happened, and he is not adept enough in this dialectic either. There is no reason to expect a radical departure of either from their respective idiosyncrasies. Both are convinced that their standpoints are obviously right. But neither is sure whether the other is right, though he is sure of the falsity of the other's view. The two work from different ideas which are mutually exclusive. Armed with scientific laws of causation and systematically tested facts the physician need not be accessible to any other idea not amenable to scientific analysis. The African, on the other hand, relies on what those before him have passed on to him, true or false, actual or mythical. But the two have a common goal which is to maintain an agreeable degree of psychosomatic equilibrium. Their major problem is the fact that they are circumspect to their social and medical circumstances. The perceived or the imagined friction between them arises precisely because the patient feels he is being manipulated from what he considers to be pertinent reality. Equally the physician suspects the patient of vacuous superstition. The result of such interaction has been near-tragedy particularly because of the colonial situation both have been working in. The scientific man is no less one dimensional than is the traditional; the physician, at best, resorts to open hostility, at worst, careless condescension. To retain his dignity, the African turns to be an arrogant impediment. And good neighborliness is as rare as ever.

III. The Colonial Era: Prospero-Caliban Situation

The relationship between the modern physician and the African traditionalist has not been peculiar to Africa. It has been the rule in all the major facets of White-Black, master-servant relationship which is the result of colonial domination by European powers. The Europeans who migrated to Africa, regardless of their status or philosophy at home looked down upon the Africans, that was the rule. The new Christian clergy who came by the same boat as the gunners set out to unseat what they regarded as the work of the devils in all their facets. In their stead, Christians intended to recreate African reality in the image of European Christianity. Politically, colonial rule destroyed the traditional geronto-cratic authority structure. To make colonial rule more effective a change in religious beliefs was deemed an asset. The missionaries were used for what they were worth, and they used the administration for their own good in their pro-selytization of the Africans. Like the missionary, the physician was able to join the band wagon since he was a patriotic member of the colonial rule. He forgot that the medical systems that existed in the past were applicable to and backed by given sociocultural correlates of their time. Problems have not been few in the transition from one sociocultural attachment to another because of such value conflicts. In the African situation, the prospero-Caliban type of relationship has been produced by the harmonious hem-ming of the native from all sides of human endeavor and the relegation of the native to the most undesirable rank in society.

How to best cope with such an idiosyncratic problem depends very much on the society concerned. Hard and fast rules would prove to be unsound regarding the optimum desired relationship between those who are in a superordinate position and those who are in a subordinate rank. In what context should the Western trained physician interact with the African? Some of the choices are quite clear. He could choose to establish a dialogue with the African by taking him as he is, a colleague, rather than as a preconceived prototype of imagination. This is perhaps better done by seeing the point of view of the patient, his expectations as well as his fears. This strategy clears the way for communi-cation and mutual respect. Another alternative is con-descension which is essentially superiority complex. Condescension has the effect of creating dependent individuals, Caliban clientele, who look more stupid than they really are. Such people are so dependent on the modern medical practitioner that what he prefers, disapproves or ignores, the dependent population uncritically acquiesces, thereby abrogating their creative potential. By design or otherwise, such is symptomatic of colonial domination. The third alternative is open hostility to the behavior, ideas and faith of the indigenous population. Force is used to legitimize desired behavior. In the 1920's in Kenya, the British colonial government and the protestant missionaries collaborated in attempts to forcefully abolish Kikuyu clitoridectomy. A Kikuyu is not fully human and certainly not a full member of the tribe unless he or she has undergone the rite of circumcision. No Kikuyu child of thirteen to eighteen years had a choice as to whether to fulfill the rite de passage or not. This extremely painful physical operation was ruled by the missionaries to be barbarous, at once cruel to human biology and at once an unchristian interference with human anatomy. To ensure that the Godly did not mix with the devils incarnate clitoridectomized girls were expelled from school for having deviated so much from the road to heaven. This open hostility helped to strengthen Kikuyu intransigence against *all* Europeans. Ever since, the saying has been "the priest and the colonial administrator are one and the same person." Not surprisingly, clitoridectomy continues to this day in some parts of the tribe. Apart from closing avenues to communication, hostility calls for further hostility on the part of the Caliban. Indeed, it is a poor method of establishing rapport suitable for a new reality.

IV. Offensives Against Traditional Medicine

In the realm of health, traditional medicine is treated with suspicion, often to an undue degree. The providers and their clients are harrassed by missionaries and other elites eager to get over the past and into the modern however relevant in the present situation. Traditional medicine has been variously labelled: sorcery, black magic, witch hunting, native superstition, any term that is able to denigrate the local population. All this is in spite of the fact that by and large traditional and modern system of medicine are perceived as different by the general population. The two systems are conceptualized not only different in their qualitative content but also in their curative approach to health maintenance. In a 1972 small rural scale survey among the Akamba people, this was shown to be the case.[11] This explains why an individual can use both systems of medicine without any feeling of contradiction since the two medical enterprises often treat different psychosomatic malfunctions. In that study it was clear that there was "Kikamba" illnesses which are only amenable to traditional forms of therapy and there are "hospital" illnesses which accordingly respond exclusively to modern medicine. Herein lies the clear non-contradictory coexistence of a supernaturally ordained etiological explanation and the modern microbial conception.

It is easier to demand that a modern physician work in the belief system of the traditional patient, quite another thing for him to appreciate the spectrum of the implications of the traditional medical conceptions.[12] It is a dilemma-ridden situation for the modern physician who has no time to think about others rather than cure diseases. If he accepts the patient as a rational man whose belief system happens to be different, ipso facto he will be legitimizing the medical logic of the indigenous patient. Fear of a boomerang effect prevents acceptance of patient beliefs. The patient might easily feel that he is not obligated to retain his ideas instead of some other new views. Would the physician be perpetuating scientifically worthless beliefs as a consequence of which he would be leading the patient into foolery? To create mutual trust between the patient and himself seems to be the only viable alternative open to the physician. Fruitful relationship with the patient is only possible when both sides appreciate their differences. The acceptance of modern scientific reasoning by the traditionalist might be a very gradual process indeed. But there is no recipe for doing it a better way. It seems pretty obvious that to deny the indigenous people a chance to show the content and quality of what they have and believe to be viable, to deny them free choice, to bulldoze them across unintelligible ideas and behavior, is tantamount to imposing new values upon them. This is what colonization of the mind is all about, enforcing irrelevant values on a society and ensuring that they are adhered to. It might well be that the modern-traditional dichotomies of disease and treatment aim at restoring self respect of the African native in response to colonial subordination.

V. Two Major Variants of the Traditional Doctor

The African traditional doctor is a blanketing term. But the concept has been defined variously. The magician, witch doctor, diviner, medicine man, herbalist, sorcerer are terms used interchangeably to refer to the traditional doctor. In essence, however, there are two varieties of traditional health experts in Africa, viz: the herbalist and the medicine man or the diviner. The dichotomy is here in reference to the Akamba ethnic group, though we believe that it is Africa-wide.

The Herbalist: A herbalist, literally, is a person who deals with herbs and herbal medicine of whatever brand concocted from selected leaves, roots or any other properties of plants. The medication thereof is explicitly for specific diseases not their underlying supernatural cause. The herbalist has the modern pharmacist as a counterpart in modern medicine. Not unlike him, he has one of the most lucrative occupations especially in an environment of countless maladies which take a heavy toll particularly among the underfives. Maternal and perinatal morbidity and mortality are common in the area, often in the same proportion as common colds. Cases of TB are invariably reported, often through the grapevine, and that such cases make deliberate attempts to avoid contact with modern medical personnel.[13] Under such "sickness" conditions a herbalist is able to scoop the financial and social rewards as a result of the demand for medical care. This demand is heavily oriented toward traditional treatment available in the locality. Low educational level of dubious quality coupled with economic backwardness contributes little or nothing to possible orientation to modern preventive medicine. The social and the harsh environmental conditions seem to sanction the operation of the herbalist in a wide ranging assortment of herbs and medicaments. The herbalist thrives because he is needed by the community.

In an area of 5 square miles, with a population of 4500, there were ten herbalists in 1973, not counting those who operated along the periphery of the location. And all of them claimed to have a sizeable number of clients. Of the ten, eight had at least three years of education in Christian Missionary schools, they were well under 45 years old. The remaining two were over 55 years old, neither had ever been to school nor ever been connected with the missionaries.

To become a herbalist, the primary requisite is empirical knowledge of herbs. A would be herbalist is expected to be able to tell the poisonous herbs from the non-poisonous ones. He is expected to know the herbs fit for external use and those fit for consumption. This knowledge is open to all male children, rarely to females. Traditionally boys were trained by their fathers, uncles, grandfathers, neighbors and so on in the art of herding livestock and hunting. In these practices plants are very important and form part of life, the herding stick, the walking stick, the arrows, spears, the tooth-brush, to name a few. This makes it imperative that those closely connected with plants understand their natural environment and their social use. On the other hand, women neither hunt nor usually herd, rather they are responsible for other more domestic chores like cooking, fetching firewood and water, weeding and the like. The emphasis on "division du travail social" among many African tribes is as preeminent as the feeling of male-female segregation! The role of women is such that they do not need herbal education. This is not to say that all male children grow up with plant knowledge "in their blood." Only a few are interested. Very few pursue an indepth study and the therapeutic potency of the plants.

The pursuit of further study may be gained through formal or informal apprenticeship to a practicing herbalist. Actually this is a rare thing. As one of the ten herbalists told me:

> Every herbalist should have inside knowledge about herbs.
> There is no secret in unused or unknown herbs. It is the
> way herbal medicine is mixed and used that varies from
> one doctor to another, the best being the one who has his
> own way of mixing herbs in such a way that the result is
> more effective than another. That is the specialist. He will
> not be eager to reveal this special expertise. He stops being
> a specialist when he has no special knowldge.

To know about herbs is to know not only the name but also
what a plant can do to the human body. It is also important
to know the strength, or the "Poison" concentration of a herb
and subsequently the illness or at least the syndrome that
will respond to the herb. Diagnostic techniques are pragmatic, not speculative. One herbalist I observed on and off
for a year insisted that the body of a human being is so
susceptible to poisonous intake that he does not experiment
on a new herb with patients, rather with his own children
and the three wives and then on relatives. He said:

> Sometimes it takes me a long time to get what I want. An
> herb I think of being good for coughing might have grown
> in the wrong soil, it might be ruined by worms. Anything
> could change it to something else. I have to test every-
> thing, individual herb by herb, then I mix one by one in
> varying quantities, tasting it every time. My three wives
> taste it too. When I have to mix five or so herbs to pro-
> duce a solution I need, it is neither interesting nor easy to
> go through the process.

There are two variants of herbalists in Kenya. The first
type consists of those who operate a "domestic clinic" to
cater for "in" or "out" patients or both, local and distant.
Usually such clinicians have other occupations besides their
medical commitment. Not unlike modern medical physicians,
these people do not advertise themselves. One of them told
me, "the effectiveness of *my* herbs speak for *me*." The
method of diagnosis in the domestic clinics reminds one of
the modern physician's diagnostic techniques and criteria.
After asking some irrelevant and routine questions—the name,
residence, distance and "what is your trouble?"—most of the
other questions asked are leading and suggestive. One would
think they are asked for effect rather than to gain insights
into the pathological or psychological state of the patient.
Like the modern physician, the herbalist seems to have made

up his mind about the illness just by looking at the patient. As a traditional surgeon, my father asks very few or no questions. He simply looks at the patient. If his seven inch hip-knife leaves the sheath, there is surgery with or without the consent of the patient. I have many times watched him perform very ghastly operations with his patients falling unconscious. He has twice operated on me. I have watched him suture up a patela in place and then send the patient to the hospital unaccompanied. The big scar on my nose reminds me of his surgical ingenuity. He stitched a young woman's eye brow and chin in place to the amazement of the village. During that surgical operation he used alcohol as a sterilizer. I have forgotten the number of times the woman collapsed and the amount of cold water poured on her to bring her to. When the medical personnel at the local clinic tried to find out who had treated her and sent her to the hospital to "prevent pus and later to remove the thread(!)," word went around the neighborhood that there was to be no talking. There was none. As to why my father asks very few questions, he retorts, "I use my eyes to think, not my head to see. When I look, I either know or do not know what to do."

The other brand of herbalists are commercial herbalists. They hawk their medicine from market to market. Often this is a full time occupation. Although these herbalists sell what they personally concoct, occasionally, they buy herbs from the clinical herbalists. Some of them have employed and apprenticed some enthusiasts to collect herbs for them and do preliminary tests, when they themselves sell and advertise their proficiency, not forgetting to mention the name of a popular clinician or diviner whenever necessary.

The commercial herbalists meet a cross section of their *ethnic* clientele and a variety of religious groups who favor different medical patterns. To cater for all and avoid scaring the noncommitted, they have in time adopted an esoteric herbal language with a remarkably exotic medical flavor characterized by small bottles, labelled and described in terms closely related to modern medicine. My observation is that small bottles signify the strength of the dose and obviously its therapeutic effectiveness. These people are all-round specialists in psychic and somatic disorders. A herbalist's popularity would diminish if he failed to have everything for everybody. The commercial herbalist may refer a customer to a diviner if necessary, not because he does not have the herb to treat but because he believes the customer's condition requires the services of a diviner, to whom we now turn.

The Diviner: A diviner or the medicine man or woman is one of the most highly regarded persons in many ethnic groups in Africa. He is also one of the chief opinion pointers.

The diviner is the religious-medical specialist who not only defines illness but also divines the circumstances of the illness. He gives the *ultimate* etiological conditions of a psychic, somatic or psychosomatic disorder, interpersonal alliances and conflicts. He is often called upon to divine community problems which might arise. The diviner is the single individual who is the community and individual consultant of sorts. He, therefore, must not only be a person of unquestionable social and moral integrity who has been accepted by other practitioners on the recommendations of the supernatural powers, but he must also dispense his duties in accordance with the age-old tribal mores ordained by the deity. The diviner is the one human being closest to God. He is, therefore, highly respected not necessarily because of what he does or has presumably achieved but for what he *is*; the interpreter of the manifestations of the spiritual and supernatural phenomena.

The diviner is equally looked up to with awe. He is a person of rather delicate emotions. If offended he could easily wreak havoc to individuals, groups or their community property. This apart, a man of his position and proximity to God is not one to be kicked around; the person who knows the cure, knows the poison and the curse too.

The religious-medical specialist can be innovative when he defines the situation and divines that certain practices ought to be or have been transgressed. His divination, community or individual, is not subject to debate. Neither could another diviner dispute a given divination. The diviner is one of the few qualified to recommend and actually order the execution of a duty, religious or value-free. He is able to cure as well as curse. Although some of what a diviner does is hidden to others, most of his activities seep out of his security and get to others who perpetuate them according to their own inclinations. The herbs and the decent services and charges the diviner offers are often adopted. His recommendations are often accepted without question mostly because of his close association with God and his intermediaries and rarely because they are any better understood. For instance, the enormous Kikuyu opposition to European rule had been ordained by a diviner, one of the most famous. During the colonial rule in Kenya and the Mau Mau rebellion, the very Christian authorities forced Kikuyu adults, all and sundry, to be ritually cleansed by diviners. They were supposed to confess their sins connected with secret and illegal oaths and to disown any membership in the organization led by Mau Mau Freedom Fighters. Ironically, confession implied that one had participated in an immoral, illegal terrorist movement and therefore, so facto, those cleansed were legally liable. Those who refused to indulge in the orgy implied their recalcitrance; they were equally liable to prosecution. But because the diviners themselves were part and parcel of the Mau Mau, they skipped some of the necessary sections in cleansing and thereby made the whole exercise null and void. For some reason, however, the cleansed and the recalcitrant eventually shared the indignity of the same detention campus the diviner did not have to endure.

The point being made here is that because of the diviner's prominent role, ascribed or achieved, real or imagined and his innovative potential, he is capable of impenetrable "conservative" force. On the one hand, he could ordain to select new behavioral components thereby legitimizing them and ensuring their adoption. For a changing society, this is desirable. New modes of life come into being dynamically with time. On the other hand, the diviner might as well be conservative when he defends the status quo. There are more diviners in the latter category than in the former.

The making of a diviner is said to begin from conception till the time he or she accepts the assumption of supernatural responsibilities. Thomas[14] has discussed the steps a would-be diviner among the Akamba passes through. One of the most well known diviners in the area told me what he had to endure before he decided to assume the holy role in 1957 after years of suffering. In his own words:

> The main work of the medicine man is to divine (kuwausya), that is to reveal the real cause of a disease. But I also heal and have been healing and divining for the last eight years. Born in 1922, I was troubled for many years. When I joined the Salvation Army Church organization my health worsened and I had to leave the Church in 1938. My health improved in a short while. In 1949, I went back to Church and my health took a nose dive into ill health. In 1956, I again left the Church. I started obeying in 1957 and was cured immediately and automatically. Obedience meant collecting the divining artifacts which are vital for treatment. This I did every day thereafter till I had all that was required of me.

> When I started obeying the ordained role, it was revealed to me in a dream that my grandmother was a diviner. During the time of the dreams I was succumbed by very deep sleep, I was sick and delirious and the dreams, which recurred for days on end, directed me where to pick the divining artifacts. Refusal to obey results in the loss of personal property, health, wives, and even life. Some seek refuge in the assumption that someone has a grudge against them and if they consult a diviner (mundu mue), they are told the real cause of their trouble. They always have to obey or face the consequences.

> How people know of the new diviner is simple. The making of a diviner is like a prophecy. People know and come to you. Those who advertise are the mercenary types, they are cheats. I am directed to use certain herbs and no others can be used however good and regardless of what I may think of a condition of a patient. Those who sell herbs (miti) in the market place are traders like any other type of trader. They are different from diviners and healers. My opinion is that the difference is the same as the difference between the modern doctor and the pharmaceutical salesman. The herbs of the salesman have no divine credibility whatever.

> To increase my repertoire of herbs, I do experiments on my own to determine the type of herb and the dosage. When I am testing a new herb, I dispense it to a few of my children to guard us from accusations of ill-will. This is the hardest part of my job, I have to put to the test what I think is right.[15]

Divining is a holy act and one cannot play or fiddle with it and stay alive. To divine is to reveal, to discover what God has forbidden or wants done. Without the right to divine, to assume this honorable responsibility, without the right to do so is sacrilegious. When I die, somebody in the family or clan will be given the responsibility. It neither dies nor leaves the clan, it is recurrent since it is divined by God himself. I am not telling you that all diviners are bona fide, you surely have crooks in your hospitals, haven't you?

The diviner went on to say that his patients come from far and wide, in the whole of the Republic. He himself travels a great deal to these areas on missions. Healing is one thing; divining is another and both do not have to be used at the same time by every patient. One patient may need herbs only, another divination alone and go elsewhere for treatment and healing.

Divination is the last resort in the process of an illness or disturbance. The client has to specifically ask for divination (as was earlier stated by a former patient). This usually occurs when the patient knows or thinks he knows of what he is suffering from. Any genuine doctor should in most cases be able to tell what disease a client has by simple examination of the circumstances that might have brought the condition about in any other person. Not all diseases, however, need divination because divination aims at the cause of the condition that is not knowable in any other way, that is answering the question why. What the malady is should not be the work of divination, this needs ordinary diagnostic techniques. As one diviner told me, "I can tell a patient what the diagnosis is, only God can tell him or her how and why the cause is." Of course most patients want to be able to connect the diagnosis with the reason or reasons of its being.

Some people go to the diviner for both divination and treatment but the numbers are decreasing. One diviner told me that many people prefer the hospital and the herbalist. Others are alienated from divination by their religious faith. Christians who go to the diviners do so at night to avoid possible stigmatization by their co-believers. This is not unusual. As recently as the 1950's, circumcised Kikuyu girls avoided publicity for fear of losing their chances of ever going to a good high school or joining a school of nursing. When discovered the girls were negatively sanctioned and their parents were removed from the annals of the Holy Communicants.

Diviners are convinced that they hold the very advanced extremities of illness control on account of being able to converse with God. The hospital doctor, said one, "uses mechanical instruments. I use my hand, something personal and human, in collaboration with divine powers to find out what is troubling the patient." Traditionally, illnesses are of three types, viz: Kikamba, European and those which are shared by both. In all there exist incurable diseases. As the diviner interviewed above said, "If I cannot cure a Kikamba illness, it is not amenable to any other treatment by a Mkamba doctor. If I fail to find the cause of an illness, another diviner if told the same story would not find the cause of the illness." This might explain the lack of competition among the diviners, they would kill each other with all sorts of witch craft and sorcery. They would spend all their time trying to protect themselves from the jealousies of their fellow diviners rather than thinking of how best to help their patients. Jealousy and evil eye, real or imaginary, are perhaps some of the most virulent aspects of African life. A case in point involved an African diviner and a modern medical doctor of European extraction. The story is related by the latter and we reproduce it at length:

> I was working in an area of lowland Machakos doing medical research on some parasitological project. The nature of my work made it necessary to treat cases which could not have come to the notice of any medical officer in the district. I lived with the people in the village. One day I woke up to find myself suffering from acute diarrhea. This was very mysterious and much more sudden that I ever knew. A villager told me that I had been bewitched by somebody and would I verify this from another diviner. I did this out of curiosity. I was told to dig round my tent and would excavate the items of bewitchment.
>
> I followed the instructions. Not far from the entrance to the tent, I excavated pieces of my own hair, what looked like parts of female genitalia, and a rat. The next day very early in the morning my fellow traditional doctor came to me suffering from malignant typhoid. He happened to be a

traditional doctor of profound experience and medical power. He confessed to me and promised that he would not repeat what he did to me. However, his pathological state responded to my prescription. Since then we have been friends and refer patients to each other. We no longer compete for clients. I find that my work has been easier ever since.[16]

Very often, though, there is little or no felt competition between the traditional doctor and the modern doctor. The latter are believed to cure only the natural (biochemical/ microbial) illnesses. Some diviners say they even refer patients to each other and to hospitals when that is necessary. They themselves go to the hospital when they contract European diseases. One diviner mentioned referrals to the hospital for X-ray and surgical purposes. Suffice it to say many more diviners neither go nor refer patients to the hospital. Diviners will insist that treatment depends on past achievement. Patients will seek the treatment they know best, not just any that comes their way. Diviners are conscientious enough not to misdirect their patients. They would like to have them go where they would get the relevant type of treatment, where they actually belong.

If a patient believes he needs a hospital injection when he actually does not, he could only be gouged out of that conviction by practical experience and demonstration that it does not work. This is the same on the case of traditional medicine. Some curative agents should not be mixed with others, but some modern medicine and traditional herbs are mixed for specific purposes.

The range of the illnesses treated by the diviner includes gastroenteritis, headaches, and the following: female diseases like lack of children, continuous menstrual flow, vaginal canal blockage and constant loss of incomplete pregnancies. Men's diseases include gonorrhea, blocked urinary canal, sexual impotency, failure to obtain lovers and so forth. Other diseases are marasmus, bilharziasis, epilepsy, skin diseases, typhoid and wounds. Three diviners said they could not cure cardiac failure, asthma and tuberculosis. They said prevention of diseases among the Akamba is impossible because people do not seek treatment unless they are sick. Moreover, what the diviner can detect are existing or perceived etiological or grass-root causes behind a given disorder. If a person comes to a diviner seeking preventive medicine he should be able to relate the reasons why he needs it. He must be suspecting somebody dead or alive or some ritual defilement or some other kind of omission. To succumb to this would render such a person culpable by others who might misinterpret the visit to the diviner. His foes might be persuaded to seek some counter medicine to thwart his evil intentions. Witchcraft accusations and counter accusations will be imminent.

It is often erroneously believed that the diviners are all capable. They are not. Their assumed all powerfulness is one of the many myths and mystics about them. A diviner related some of his experiences in his profession of more than 25 years:

> I can help to make measles develop more quickly, then subsequently cure it. But when the disease has made a child so ill and helpless, it is useless to come to me. The child will die any way.
>
> Occasionally with some luck, I have been able to treat and cure a child brought to me half dead. It takes me only three or four hours to treat a serious but not desparate condition whose treatment has to be very careful and intensive.
>
> There was this child dying of measles. It took me a few hours to cure him. I gave him strong doses of *my* herb, massaged him thoroughly and the big elongated reddish worm was emitted anally from the belly. There upon, he was able to sit down on his own. The boy and the parents went home that day.
>
> Except for one woman, old and already worn out by age, I have never treated anybody who later died or died during therapy.[17]

That particular diviner-cum-herbalist said the cause of measles, pertussis and acute diarrhea are similar. They are caused by a reddish brown worm lodged in the stomach just under the spleen. This is the ordinary or the natural cause. But the ultimate cause is another; that is, these childhood diseases could spring from varying causes. Evil men, for instance, or the negation of socio-religious obligation may result in one or two diseases. Those who bear a grudge against others are likely to curse or use fetish power to cause harm on whomever they like. The fetish could result in any of the diseases.

To treat, or more appropriately, to heal, the resultant illness, the sick needs a similar magical power to counter the fetish cast by the assailant. Usually when a fetish has been cast by a female witch doctor a counter fetish is sought from a female. Some diseases though defined by male or female diviners require sex-specific healers, males for male illnesses, females for female malfunctions.

The foregoing section of the diviner culminates in the following conclusions:

(1) That to divine is a holy, sacred or spiritual calling performed by a supernaturally ordained person on the request of another person seeking socioeconomic and sociospiritually "competent help";

(2) That divination is a gift of rare spiritual power to apprehend, to reveal, the malpractices of man against man, the man against the social order;

(3) That divination verifies the fear of the needy of competent help that man is essentially evil;

(4) That one needs to guard against the evils of man and against personal sins of omissions and commissions with special powers dispensable only by a few;

(5) That there are illnesses which have two causes, crudely put, the immediate or the natural, and the ultimate or the supernatural. The latter demands divination for the purpose of healing or as Ackernecht[18] says:

> ...There are many well testified cases in primitive tribes where magic kills by suggestion. ...Why should the power that kills not be able to heal? The medicine man is a soul doctor and his fellow primitive. . .needs him badly. . . .His rigid system which ignores doubt, dispels fear, restores confidence, and inspires hope.

VI. Philosophies and History

That there are many herbalists and religious-medical specialists in many african societies is not at issue. Neither is the fact that these two did not start operating to oppose the establishment of the new medicine questioned. But some might question the thesis that the contemporary religious, social, medical and economic structure intensified the co-existence of both the modern and the traditional medical services.

The historical situation indemnified those who argue like Leighton that "changing a people's customs is an even delicate responsibility than surgery."[19] The religious groups and their colonial background forgot that it is no mean task to change a society. They simply wanted to ensure that the new society in which they worked would be a carbon copy of their own in matters of faith. They ignored the foundations of the new faith and whatever was before their arrival. An impasse in exchange of ideas was created precisely because the new and the old did not understand each other. The confusion and suspicion that followed entrenched the traditional medical services against the onslaught of what was considered by the indigenous populations as a "blind-end" medical practice perpetuated by a sacrilegious group. The new medicine was a blind-end because the people did not understand it. The little they did was devoid of the ideas of ultimate cause. It cured only the obvious and left the immense core basically untouched. It was a somatic therapy conforming to some of its tenets especially along a body-mind dualism. The modern medical personnel were sacrilegious in the eyes of the people because they set aside or banished the indigenous religious faiths and banned their behavioral concomitants. Jomo Kenyatta[20] put it thus:

> ...Christian religion in Africa did not take into account...
> the communal life of the African regulated by customs
> and traditions handed down from generation to generation.
> They failed too to realize that...all the members of a
> tribe...were bound up as one organic whole and con-
> trolled by an iron-bound code of duties. The agencies of
> Western religious bodies, when they arrived in Africa, set
> about to tackle problems which they were not trained for.
> They condemned customs and beliefs which they could
> not understand.

The absolute lack of compromise between old and new religions in Africa helps to explain the reason why the herbalist and the diviner are still very important person-alities. Many of them have used this to argue that they are more efficacious in treatment than modern medicine, which is only based on their warped and faceless reasoning. But the point is that the new medicine was never understood by the people who are supposed to use it. So the would-be clients turn around and say it is no good. One of the fundamentals of changing behavior is familiarity and education, and these are today far from enough in many parts of the continent. The patronage of traditional medicine seems to have been engendered by a fight-response to the new medicine. Today the perceived hostility-drama is often much less nonexistent and often flows the other direction towards modern medical personnel and their practice.

In the realm of preventive medicine modern medicine contradicts traditional conceptions of disease etiology. It is here that modern science contradicts traditional science, if we take science to be a body of knowledge systematically deduced from conditions and observations of a people. Preventive medicine expounds on the scientific causal factors and how these could effectively be controlled. The traditional man, on the other hand, finds this either a semantic contradiction or pitiable ignorance on the part of modern medical conceptions. Traditionally, the immediate cause of disease may have any shape and description but ultimately the "why me" question dramatically personified etiology. There may be a juxtaposition of sophisticated explanatory strategies why what happened had to happen the way it did and to the recipeint in particular. The modern medical practitioner often commits the error of complacency, congratulating himself for being so profound and far-sighted without ever knowing that his explanatory variables are primarily and inextricably biomedical, microbial and bacteriological phenomena or in general they are based on natural causality. They are irrelevant to the native African. He sees the ultimate causes as phychosocial agents invested in man. This ultimate causality states that whatever misfortune befalls man it must have been caused by another man or by personal omission of some ritual. This questions the fundamental basis of germ theory. And the query is philosophical. The African wants to know the reason why on earth should a small "insect" like the fly, cause discomfort to man and his family and wealth. Why should such a minute creature want to harm a man with whom there is nothing in common? They have no common land boundary. There is no envy on the part of the small creature that the man is more wealthy or that he is a celebrated local jurist. If the insect is said to have caused the illness, then it must have been sent by somebody, by a cultural being envious of the culprit's well being!

Not that the traditional causal explanations deny the existence of microbial cases of infections. On the contrary, they attribute them to man. What the African theorist says is that the modern medical concepts are only half the truth, and half truths are by and large idiosyncratic, wrong or down right nonsensical. His explanatory variables are intertwined with his cultural past and present whereas the modern notions relegate this to irrelevant sociopsychological innuendos bordering on illogical interpretations of natural phenomena. The African thinking on disease prevention begins from man that he is socially and necessarily evil and then concludes with other natural phenomena. He will not prevent the disease as such rather he will protect himself from being bewitched by others or will protect himself from others by betwitching them and thereby ward off any ill omen that might come to him otherwise.

To fully appreciate this facade of African traditional medical practice, modern medical personnel have first to penetrate the African cultural-religious cosmological struccture.[21] This is no mean task.[22] Indeed, it is so intrinsic to the African mind and organization that much of preventive modern medicine has been accepted as a matter of convenience rather than through conviction. The fact that preventive medicine takes time to bear fruit makes it even more difficult to convince the African or its efficacy. As a consequence there is an immense popularity for therapeutic medicine which should ordinarily be secondary to preventive health as a potential for health promotion in a pre-literate community.

Yet it is this social, cultural, and religious structure that modern medicine is expected to pierce through, both directly and indirectly, by modern formal education. In those areas where formal education is well advanced, it has not proved to be capable of setting aside the myths and mystics of the philosophy of traditional medicine with all that it entails. On the one hand, the modern physician has not tried to understand the traditional doctor. On the other, the traditional doctor is suspicious of the modern physician who is part of the power structure and who has often colluded with the government to oust the traditional doctor. Again there is simply no common base for dialogue in medical matters. The scientific and the nonscientific are hypothesizing from radically different points about very diverse points of view. The validity of an argument is a matter of consistency, not of truth. Although contradictions in an argument cannot be sustained, causal connection in a disease etiology is a different matter from logical connection. Traditional beliefs are scrapped to bolster up the use of either traditional or modern medicine, the latter on a trial and error basis. This being the case, we are led to believe that when scientific medical beliefs exist side by side with the nonscientific, the potential efficacy of both is radically reduced. But as long as the two systems of medicine are functionally perceived as different and exclusive alternatives, this fear might be removed. But just as too many cooks spoil the broth, too many doctors with most probably varying disgnoses, treatments, and prognoses might be inconsequential to a patient.

But alas, there is a glaring paradox. As far as the African patient is concerned the quality of one system depends on the type of illness at hand. Modern medicine is at times as irrelevant as the traditional medicine is in respect to some diseases. When one system is called for, it is expected to be effective whether through magic, virtue or science does not matter. Sometimes one is an alternative to the other. The duality of the two systems is clearly established. But the poverty of many African countries is an added inhibiting factor to the practice of modern medicine; the necessarily basic apparatus are missing and other facilities are either inadequate or just absent. Because the patients are out of proportion to the physician population, any attempt to practice ideal modern health services remains a far cry whatever the patient may think. The poverty reverberates in the hue and cry against the use of modern medicine when a relative dies in the hospital. If what is practiced in the hospital in the poor countries is only the basic health provision with little or no relationship to modern medicine in the Western world, it is in point to doubt whether it can be competitive to traditional medicine. It is a poor competitor since the traditional transcends the basic. To get the benefit of both, it is more useful to educate and incorporate traditional doctors into modern medicine to use them as vehicles of change rather than antagonists. Ignoring and harassing them, as is the case today, is banishing traditional medicine to its natural self-propagating cocoon where it is further entrenched to the detriment of the health improvement and modernization potential of the indigenous populations.

REFERENCES

[1]Mburu, F. M.: Traditional and Modern Medicine Among the Akamba Ethnic Group, unpublished M.A. thesis, Makerere University, Kampala, 1973, p. 57.

[2]*Ibid.*, p. 59.

[3]Ndeti, K.: "Sociocultural Aspects of Tuberculosis Defaultation: A Case Study," *Social Science and Medicine*, 6:397-412 (June, 1972).

[4]Mburu, F. M., *op. cit.*

[5]Bloom, S. W.: *The Doctor and His Patient*, New York, 1963, p. 158.

[6]Mburu, F. M., *op. cit.*, p. 58.

[7]Mungai, J.M.: "The Anthropological Basis of Medicine in East Africa," *African Scientist*, 2:77-84, 1970.

[8]Twumasi, P.A.: "Ashanti Traditional Medicine," *Transition*, 41:50-65, 1972.

[9]Mburu, F. M., *op. cit.*, p. 60.

[10]Dubos, R.: *Man, Medicine and Environment*, New York, 1970, p. 97.

[11]Mburu, F. M.: Education, Illness and Health in an Area of Machakos District, Mimeo, Medical Research Center, Nairobi, 1972.

[12]Luijk, N. N. van: Medical Sociological Research in the Machakos District, Kenya Mimeo, Medical Center Nairobi, 1972.

[13]Ndeti, K., *op. cit.*

[14]Thomas, A. E.: Adaption to Modern Medicine in Lowland Machakos, Kenya, Ph.D. dissertation, Stanford University, 1970.

[15]Mburu, F. M., *op. cit.*, p. 76.

[16]*Ibid.*, p. 135.

[17]*Ibid.*, p. 97.

[18]Ackernecht, E.H.: Problems of Primitive Medicine, *Bulletin of the History of Medicine*, Vol. II, p. 513-514, 1942.

History of Medicine, Vol. II, p. 513-514, 1942.

19Leighton, A. H. in *Human Problems in Technological Change*, by Spicer, E. H. (ed.), John Wiley & Sons, New York, 1967, p. 16.

20Kenyatta, Jomo: *Facing Mount Kenya*, Secker and Warburg, London, 1938, pp. 270-271.

21Ndeti, K: The Relevance of African Traditional Doctor in Scientific Medicine, Mimeo, Department of Sociology, University of Nairobi, 1968.

22————: Elements of Akamba Life, Ph.D. Dissertation, Syracuse University, 1967.

INDIGENOUS HEALING

Ruth G. Dawkins and A.B. Dawkins, Jr.

People have been struggling for many years over the issue of what constitutes mental illness. A very general definition has emerged and it goes something like this—every society has some structure of values and mores. The people of the society learn these from various institutions—family, religion, education and government. When an individual or a group of individuals become deviants to the structure, he or they are analyzed and are placed in appropriate levels of different categories of mental illness. Since a society needs its people or else it wouldn't be a society, it then goes about creating professions, careers and jobs so that the society may be preserved—not the people, but the society. When the society is spoken of, it is spoken of in the same impersonal way that the government is spoken of. It is a word, an institution, a structure, but not people. So, when we speak of mental illness, we already assume, based on its definition, that the structure of our society is correct. Therefore deviants are criminals or mentally ill or both. It is easy to be both since the same method is used to judge both—a person's actions and thinking as related to the rules and regulations of society as interpreted by the so-called recognized authorities of that society who have been taught via the various institutions what to think and not how to think. If their word is not accepted and respected then we have the other built-in punishments—God will not love you and you'll go to hell. To prove this, God is set up to sanction the court system (In God We Trust), the capitalistic system, the government, the medical institutions, etc., etc. God's blessings are even brought to bear in the gory but "glorious" business of sending planes off to bomb and kill thousands upon thousands of people and other living things. Obviously and indeed, if *The Deity* sanctions the values of a system, the deviants of that system must be insane.

Judging from the geographical locations of most comprehensive mental health centers with rather large staffs of mental health personnel, the bulk of the insanity in America lies in the low socio-economic communities alias the ghettoes, and more recently labeled "culturally deprived," "melting pot," "poverty" and now "war zone." That's right! The government declared war on it, and one regiment of soldiers sent in to fight this war was the mental health personnel. This is justified because research shows that one of the direct casualties of poverty is mental illness. Where else but in the ghettoes of this country would they send the systemized structured mind of psychiatrists, psychologists, sociologists, social workers, etc., etc., in a massive police onslaught to cool out the struggle, their sole purpose to manipulate, exploit, divide, confuse and if these methods are not successful on the black people, there is always the pulls mental institutions which are political prisons and naturally the 38 white solution to black problems. All approved of by the ruling class of this country and the poor pays for this mental genocide under another guise called personal income tax. The PFCs in this regiment were the so-called non-professional mental health workers, now intellectually referred to as "indigenous healers." Immediately the system, with their left wing, opportunistic, radical revolutionary, reactionaries, coopted the whole scene by presenting an accepted label,— "indigenous healing." To top the whole rotten scene and to cover the rip off, they use the opportunistic third world people who are nothing but oreo cookies to front for them. Indigenous healing is not new. Only the acceptable label is new. It's a skill as old as man, that deals with complementing man's heaviest struggle—the freedom of his mind and body from all oppressive forces. Whenever this skill was discovered by European man, who is hell bent on imposing his subjective values, one of which is his innate superiority which he insists gives him the rights of ownership over all, he armed himself with his God's blessings and stole and killed and took all he could understand, for his personal gains. That which he could not understand and therefore could not deal with (truth, vibrations and love, which he called magic or witchcraft) he drove underground or tried to destroy with violence and Christianity. Evil couldn't know that you cannot destroy truth. History tells the story—Africa, Asia, South America,

187

North America, etc. Through all this, "indigenous healing" is still alive and very effective.

Traditional psychiatry, after the sick man Freud, again came to the forefront of the world off the blacks of the Hollywood actors and actresses who fell for the game that analysis by the structured psychiatric mind, would make them a better person and maybe a human being. A great deal of money was made during this fad, but it became necessary to move into other areas of manipulation and exploitation (in the name of progress). Naturally the only other provider of substantial amounts of monies in gross is the poor.

For years psychiatry was something the poor never heard of (in the South Bronx, 40 years) and they were brainwashed to feel that mental illness was something disgraceful (the only name they knew for mental illness was crazy) not only to them but also to their family, so regardless of how they felt, they dare not get mentally ill because that was taboo, but they survived. Now all of a sudden there is a mad rush to the ghettoes of these vultures, dripping with guilt, racism, elitism and all other types of isms, trying to shed their sick loads on the poor as if the poor did not already have an extremely heavy load called *poverty* and some of them had to add being *black* to it.

These frustrated people poured into the ghettoes of Amerikka with all types of mental health programs willing and able with their medications to help the oppressed people suffer peacefully. With their madness and their whiteness, loaded with all types of tranquilizing drugs, they swarmed on the third world people giving them pills and false hopes that through their systematized white-oriented therapy, black people will become well and maybe get an opportunity to move into the mainstream of white Amerikka. This is all part of the white economy trip, and the guilt ridden ones try to palm off pills, forms, waiting and the right to suffer peacefully, as the way to fight the social ills of this capitalistic country. Others, who have accepted the phony elitist position that the system has provided for them get caught up in other separations, that prove for them their elitism. We now rap about the "*providers*" and "*consumers*" of health. This is a contradiction that constantly has to be clarified not only to the poor but to the petty fools who are hung into the label bag. Let us look at it realistically. The oppression that the system brings down on the masses is so great, that if they are not geared to deal with it, they fall apart mentally and physically. Therefore, through oppression and repression the masses are the providers of ill health and the systematized thinking health professional becomes the vulturistic consumer. Case in point: there is a "doctor" in the south-east Bronx (ghetto) who made a million and a half dollars in one year—a patient every seven to twelve minutes. Question: who is the provider and who is the consumer?

The white system trained health professionals and white people have never been able to identify or relate to the problems of the third world people. If not because of their racism or whitism, it is through their madness that some of them have not been awakened as yet to the fact that they have been living under a false premise—their superiority. Their conditioning in medical school and resident training has geared them to remove themselves from people, with the false idea that if they do not identify or relate they will be able to look at the patient and the patient's problems objectively. So the whole concept of traditional psychiatry is based on negativism. When they saw the downfall of psychiatry and the rise of grassroots healing, they quickly coopted the movement by labeling it community mental health. It is amazing how frightened these agents of the system become when they have to face reality. That is that neither the system's pills nor its politics are doing much to change society's ills, and there is a definite undercurrent of something else going on among our "sick" grassroots population which is giving them back the sanity they once had. They are gaining the consciousness they need to place the real madness in its proper perspective. This is coming from the masses—the majority of the people in this so-called democratic society. The masses, who were referred to as "beasts" by one of the founding pirate fathers of this country. He knew he was right because he helped create it.

Instead of checking out and positively dealing with the reason for this new attitude among the people they should be serving, they give in to their fright and greed and resort to such devious methods of retaining their power as cooptation through conferences, and papers written with the aid of grass roots health workers. They give the worker the false feeling that their work will be recognized and their methods will be incorporated into the system. At the same time, programs and laws are created that limit the worker and prevent him from using workable solutions. This is supported by federal and local governments whose vulturistic reactionaries use their credentials as controlling factors to discredit or fire those who are a threat to their existence as vultures. When this fails because now the struggle is being taken to the streets by the revolutionary health worker, the professional organizations with the aid of the system then eliminates the health programs within the ghetto areas through legal cutbacks and after awhile eliminates the program completely.

We have to constantly deal with reality, because herein lies the growth of our people, so we come to another case in point: Dr. Joe English, formerly head of the National Institute of Mental Health, now head of one of the most reactionary organizations in health, receives approximately $67,000 in salary per year. It is rumored around the hospitals that he works approximately twenty hours per week, is the last "doctor" on earth you will see in the emergency room in the ghetto on the weekends when more than ever there is a need for competent doctors. This man sits in his very beautiful office somewhere in the business district of downtown Manhattan and makes policies concerning the health of poor people. One year's salary plus expenses would provide better health care for 100,000 people in the South Bronx for one year. This same man is a product of the racist, elitist medical colleges who send their butchers into the butcher shops called ghetto hospitals. While they are there for four years experimenting (interning), they maim and kill. Some even pretend they are radical for that period of time and as soon as their four years are up they fly, leaving the door open for the medical empire to send in a fresh batch of butchers. They come and they leave a trail of dead behind them with their experiments and malpractice, no knowledge shared but one— the poor is there to be experimented on or obey orders without questioning. Workers are not even permitted to question the deaths of their brothers and sisters. This part comes under the label of confidentiality.

It has now been realized that there is a very important portion of the art of healing that cannot be taught because as yet it cannot be scientifically broken down and categorized. Once it has been given the acceptable label, it can now be measured or looked at empirically. That's where we are now with the science of: Mental Health, category: *"Indigenous Healing."* We could continue breaking down the economic, political, racist, cooptive approach to traditional and now indigenous healing of the poor, we could even include more examples that bring the light to the "mentally ill," but we don't want to get ahead of science and its system and its structured method of investigation.

Indigenous healing is the cooptation of the third world people's methods of dealing with the sick in the low income community. Since it is so important to science to be able to label, categorize and sub-categorize, here is an overview of about six types of "indigenous healers." Bear in mind that this is the beginning of a categorical hell that will grow not because of its acceptance, but in spite of it.

1. *The Opportunistic Indigenous Healer*

One who believes in the mainstream of American society—but for himself, and social climbs through the mental health field on the backs of the people. He comes across as a ghetto authority to all those in higher positions (his masters) who cannot or (in 1972) dare not dispute him. This type may or may not also hold "credentials," be one of the so-called minority races and is usually sure of his leadership of the people. He writes superintellectual papers on *his* theories, *his* achievements, *his* conclusions, etc., etc. He will befriend anyone who seemingly "knows the ropes" and famous names of people either in the professional authoritative ranks or among the "leaders" of the lower echelon of the masses and has a fair knowledge of the language used by both. He is able to act out any role i.e., professional, cultural, nationalist, revolutionary, reactionary, etc., when it is beneficial to him.

2. *Semi-Opportunistic Types*
   Fears and respects the professional in the field. Believes in the mainstream society for both himself and the people he serves. Jobs and better living conditions is the answer and he believes that this can be attained by all with his help through the system.

3. *Pacifist Type Indigenous Healer*
   Usually is a great believer in one of the systems accepted religions and leaves all solutions to problems and healing up to God, the professionals and the Great White Fathers in Washington. He collects his salary every payday religiously, and takes no risks i.e., job, status, counter-system opinions, etc., etc. All three of these categories fall for the sweat shop psychiatric game.

4. *Cultural Nationalist Indigenous Healer*
   Usually, of the petty bourgeoisie capitalist type who uses color, race, national or cultural backgrounds, etc. to inspire the masses, yet keep themselves in the foreground to achieve position, salary, ego, prestige. Yet he is essential to bring the masses through certain hazardous paths to the freedom road but deserts them in the face of direct confrontation. Without his knowledge, he has become the pawn of the system in one of its oldest games—the divide and conquer routine.

5. *Soul Therapist—Indigenous Healer*
   One whose mind has been liberated to the point where he is constantly shedding useless intellectually learned values and leaves himself open to the feel or field of environmental vibrations. He has experienced each of the aforementioned levels of growth and many not mentioned here. He has used each experience as a catalyst for growth for himself and his people. Uses his own method of analysis, methods that are apolitical to the system. Experiences some fear but nevertheless risks status, money and sometimes his life for the health and freedom of his people.

6. *Revolutionary Health Worker*
This worker is the health worker who knows that the only psychology needed for the freedom of black people is guns and revolution. This worker therefore contributes to the mental health and health of his people through his practices and deeds. He makes but one statement to the cooptive system in terms of his methodology: "Those who tell do not know: those who know do not tell."

When people are aware of how mental illness and ill health is caused by oppression and slavery and can deal with it adequately, not for individual freedom, but a collective freedom, then the need for the so-called professional will be eliminated, for then solutions will be derived at on a collective basis which is part of black people's (by black is meant all people of color) history and culture.

AMERICAN LEGAL AND POLICY
IMPLICATIONS OF TRADITIONAL HEALING

John H. Shepherd, Esq.

This chapter is concerned with the legal and public policy implications of herbal medicine or traditional healing, which will be referred to as "unconventional medicine" in contradistinction to what the conventional wisdom recognizes as the practice of medicine. We will not be discussing the validity or invalidity of unconventional medicine's concepts but rather the approaches which one might expect legislatures and courts to take when confronted with its practice or its advocacy.

It will be instructive to begin with a case decided by the Michigan Supreme Court in 1926, *People of the State of Michigan* v. *Banks*. The defendant Frank S. Banks was convicted of illegally practicing medicine under a statute which provided as follows:

> Any person who shall practice medicine or surgery in this state or who shall advertise in any form or hold himself or herself out to the public as being able to treat, cure or alleviate human ailments or diseases and who is not the lawful possessor of a certificate or registration or license. . . shall be deemed guilty of a misdemeanor. . .it shall be the duty of the prosecuting attorneys of the counties of this state to prosecute violations of the provisions of this act. . . .This act shall not apply. . .to persons who confine their ministrations to the sick or afflicted to prayer and without the use of material remedies. . . .In this act, unless otherwise provided, the term "practice of medicine" shall mean the actual diagnosing, curing or relieving in any degree, or professing or attempting to diagnose, treat, cure or relieve any human disease, ailment, defect or complaint, whether of physical or mental origin, by attendance or by advice, or by prescribing or furnishing any drug, medicine, appliance, manipulation or method, or by any therapeutic agent whatsoever.

The evidence at the trial disclosed that the defendant lived in a home in the city of Lansing, Michigan; that there was a large sign in front of his house on which was painted the word "Banks"; that in his house was a room designated by a sign "waiting room" from which a door led into another room designated "office"; that in this room the defendant conferred with people who called upon him and in it were a number of tables with bottles similar to bottles of medicine.

One Roy French and his brother Elno went to the defendant's office in May of 1924. Roy told the defendant that he was suffering with "tuberculosis of the bone," that he had had an operation on his hip and that there was a hole in it. Banks told the brothers that he "could cure that." He said, "that his medicine would soak down into them holes in that bone and drive the poison out of his system;" and that "patients that he got was mostly people that had been to doctors and the doctors could not cure them so he got lots of patients that way."

Roy French purchased a bottle of medicine from Banks for which he paid $25.00 (in 1926!).

Banks recommended to Roy French that the medicine only had to be used once and that it could be injected in the hip and that afterwards if there were any other infections in his body the skin over it would turn colored. Further instructions were given to keep the affected area wet from six to eight hours with "the cancer medicine." Other advice was given to Roy over a period of weeks during which time Roy's legs and face became swollen and marked changes in color in his face occurred. Banks gave an opinion to Roy that the poison had come to the surface and that he was glad because he was now confident of curing him.

The Michigan Supreme Court found no difficulty in determining that Banks had been engaged in the practice of medicine without a license and the conviction was upheld. Bank's attorney insisted that no diagnosis had been made and that the selling of medicine was not engaging in the practice of medicine within the inhibition of the statute. The defendant did not call himself a doctor nor did he hold himself out to the public as such and he made no physical examination of Roy. He simply took his word as to the nature of his ailment. However, the Court stated that he did undertake to treat the ailment and sold him medicine giving specific instructions as to the manner in which the remedy should be applied. The Court added:

> Many doctors at times prescribe medicines for patients relying on their statements as to the nature of their ailments

and without making a diagnosis thereof. The charge for
the bottle of medicine was out of proportion to its value
as such. It is apparent that it included a fee to the defendant
for the service rendered by him in prescribing it.

The Court further indicated that the totality of the
evidence tended to prove that the defendant was not simply
selling medicines but was professing to treat and cure human
ailments. The Court concluded that, "that which defendant
did warranted the submission of the case to the jury and
justified the verdict rendered."

It is of enormous significance to the analysis of this
chapter that the Court, in a criminal case does not request
the jury to determine what happened so that the Court might
determine whether the facts found by the jury constitute the
offense (e.g. the practice of medicine) within the meaning of
the statute. The trial court in the Banks case submitted to the
jury the question of whether the basically undisputed facts
constituted the practice of medicine and the Supreme Court
simply concluded that from all of the evidence which was
available, the jury (i.e. the community) was justified in concluding that the defendant had been practicing what the jury
understood to be "medicine." The defendant Banks became
a criminal therefore because twelve people taken from a cross
section of his community determined that what he was doing
fit into their notion of what medical practitioners usually do.
In upholding the conviction, the Supreme Court said that the
trial Court was justified in permitting the jury to make this
evaluation and that there was enough evidence to support the
jury's conclusion. The real judge in this case was the totality
of the community's experience, collective wisdom, pre-
judices, preconceived ideas and good faith conclusions as to
what is right and what is wrong. Had this totality of
experience not been imbedded in the minds of the jurors in
the particular configuration which was present in Michigan
in 1926, those same jurors might have concluded that what
Banks was doing was good for the community and they
might have concluded that he was not practicing medicine,
that he did not have to obtain a license and that he was not
guilty of the offense charged.

The Banks case is an illustration of the concept that

acts are rendered criminal because they are done under circumstances in which the community believes they will probably cause some harm which the law ought to attempt to prevent and the test of criminality which the jury applies is the degree of danger which the jury believes accompanies that act under all of the surrounding circumstances. The jury is asked by the Court to find whether the defendant has practiced medicine but their result is determined by their conception of whether the defendant's acts were wrong or harmful.

What constitutes the practice of medicine will vary from state to state and from time to time and will depend upon an almost infinite number of variables including the composition of the legislature, the conservative versus liberal attitudes of the courts, the power of organized medicine, the influence of religious institutions or consumer protection groups and the ambitions or diligence of prosecuting attorneys. A state may, in the exercise of its power to regulate conduct for the general health, safety and welfare, adopt legislation which regulates and defines the practice of medicine and all states in the United States have done so. Most statutes do not clearly define what shall constitute a violation; instead they use general definitions prohibiting the practice of medicine without a license and therefore the problems raised in the Banks case in Michigan have general applicability throughout the country. As a general rule one may conclude that unless a practitioner is qualified by license he ought not to deal with disease or wounds in any manner and he is running the risk of being found to be practicing medicine if he is caught and prosecuted. It is true that there have been exceptions to this rule and that persons have occasionally been able to avoid criminal responsibility by establishing that they were simply selling herbs without becoming involved in prescribing their use but these exceptions are rare and one proceeds at his own risk. The risk is that a prosecutor will decide to test to the question of whether the acts complained of constitute the practice of medicine and that a jury using the rationale of the Banks case will agree that they do.

The problems of analysis which are present in the context of a criminal case are equally present in civil matters where the question is not whether one is guilty of a crime but whether the defendant must pay damages to a plaintiff who has been injured by a practitioner of unconventional medicine. In a civil proceeding the defendant is asked only to pay money and the jury, often believing that there is insurance, is normally not concerned that its verdict will impose undue harm upon the defendant in proportion to the harm which has been done to the plaintiff. Some of the theories of civil liability which can be invoked against a practitioner of unconventional medicine can be stated briefly and in each of them the ultimate question is likely to be the same. "Has the defendant committed an act which in the best judgment of a cross section of the community constitutes a harm which needs to be punished, prevented or compensated?" These theories are:

BREACH OF WARRANTY—The sale of herbs is the sale of goods and in almost every state there exists under the law an implied warranty by the seller that the goods are fit for the use intended. An injured plaintiff will sue the seller for breach of warranty and the seller will defend himself by claiming that the scope of the warranty was extremely limited given the ambiguous representations which may have been made at the time of sale; that there was no breach of warranty because the herbs were fit for the purpose intended and that the plaintiff did not follow directions; that the injury caused to the plaintiff was not the result of taking the herbs but rather some other causal connection is to be found. Whatever the arguments on either side one can expect that a jury faced with facts similar to the Banks case will return a verdict in favor of the plaintiff regardless of the persuasiveness of the various arguments put forward by the defense.

FRAUD—The plaintiff will argue that the defendant made fraudulent representations concerning the efficacy of the unconventional treatment and that the plaintiff parted with his money under false representations resulting in his physical and pecuniary damage. The same jury which sat in the Banks case would not have any difficulty in finding that Banks was guilty of fraud and that he should pay damages to an injured plaintiff. In all civil cases the Court would inquire whether with reasonable diligence the defendant could have foreseen the danger and again, using the preceding analysis, juries will have little difficulty in finding that the defendant failed to exercise reasonable care under all of the circumstances.

MEDICAL MALPRACTICE—A licensed medical practitioner using unconventional medical preparations or techniques may escape criminal prosecution but he is not immune from a civil action for malpractice. The law imposes a duty upon a physician to use reasonable skill and care for the safety and well-being of his patient and he is liable to the patient for an injury resulting from an absence of the requisite knowledge and skill or the omission to use reasonable care and diligence. The question which the Court asks is whether the practitioner has applied a degree of care or skill which is ordinarily employed by the profession generally under similar conditions and in like surrounding circumstances. A physician is required to possess that reasonable degree of learning, skill and experience which ordinarily is possessed by others in his profession and he must exercise reasonable and ordinary care in the exercise of his skill taking into account the reasonable and ordinary care, skill and diligence practiced by physicians in good standing in the same area, in the same general line of practice and under similar circumstances.

In determining a course of treatment a physician is required to exercise reasonable care and the propriety of his treatment in any given case is normally determined with reference to all of the pertinent facts in existence which were known or which should have been known in the exercise of such reasonable care. On this rationale, physicians have been held liable for an injury resulting to the patient from the mistaken administration of the wrong drug or medicine and here also the question of liability will probably be determined with reference to the threshold question of whether the jury believes that the use of unconventional medical techniques which have not been tested by conventional methods is a harm or a wrong which requires some form of redress. The theory of liability is largely irrelevant. The question is whether those with power (juries, judges, legislators, the A.M.A.) believe that something needs to be done.

A somewhat peripheral (but frequently practical) consideration is that of the difficulty which will exist in obtaining insurance to protect against law suits arising out of the practice of unconventional medicine. The field of products liability is mushrooming and insurance companies will be reluctant to write insurance policies covering the dispensing of herbal medicine by unlicensed practitioners. Licensed physicians, already burdened by increasing insurance rates, may find exclusions written into their policies absolving the insurance company of liability for injuries arising out of the practice of unconventional medicine and they may find their policies cancelled in the event that they are sued for injuries arising out of unconventional practices. The current medical malpractice controversy which exists throughout the country is not likely to increase the risk-taking propensities of a physician concerned with making a living and staying out of court.

The purpose of this chapter has not been to deal with every conceivable legal issue which can arise in the practice of unconventional medicine but rather it has been to focus the reader's attention on the analytical process which is used (and which will be used in the future) in determining whether any given course of conduct will be permitted. The conclusion is inevitable that it is the conscience of the community (as defined by the community) which will control. If any new method of treatment is to become accepted it will first have to run the gauntlet of the medical power structure and be subjected to whatever empirical testing is deemed to be appropriate by those in command of the reins of medical authority. Certain unconventional medical practices may become the conventional wisdom of another day. Others will be discarded either with justification or without it. Has it ever been otherwise?

One might ask whether this relativism and the willingness to let community standards control the outcome of criminal cases are anachronisms or whether the courts might be willing to go beyond ephemeral local tastes and set standards of their own. I would conclude that not much has changed since 1926 and the Banks case and, in support of this conclusion, I would cite the case of Miller v. The State of California decided by the United States Supreme Court in 1973. The Defendant was tried by jury and was convicted of violating the California Penal Code by knowingly distributing obscene matter. The brochures in question contained pictures and drawings very explicitly depicting men and women engaging in a variety of sexual activities. The Court recognized that states have a legitimate interest in prohibiting dissemination or exhibition of obscene material when the mode of dissemination carries with it a significant danger of offending the sensibilities of unwilling recipients or of exposure to juveniles. Chief Justice Burger acknowledged that no majority of the Court has at any given time been able to agree on a standard to determine what constitutes obscene, pornographic material subject to regulation under the police power of the states. However, he stated that it has been categorically settled by the Court that obscene material is unprotected by the freedom of speech provisions of the first Amendment to the Constitution. These Amendments, says Burger, have never been treated as absolutes and "in resolving the inevitably sensitive questions of fact and law, we must continue to rely on the jury system, accompanied by the safeguards that Judges, rules of evidence, presumption of innocence, and other protective features provide, as we do with rape, murder and a host of other offenses against society and its individual members."

Rather than give the jury explicit guidelines to follow in determining guilt or innocence Burger says (in a 5-4 opinion with a vigorous dissent by Justice Douglas):

> Under a National Constitution, fundamental First Amendment limitations on the powers of the states do not vary from community to community, but this does not mean that there are, or should or can be, fixed, uniform national standards of precisely what appeals to the 'prurient interest' or is 'patently offensive.' These are essentially questions of fact, and our Nation is simply too big and too diverse for this Court to reasonably expect that such standards could be articulated for all 50 states in a single formulation even assuming the prerequisite consensus exists. When triers of fact are asked to decide whether the average person applying contemporary community standards would consider certain materials prurient, it would be un-

> realistic to require that the answer be based on some abstract formulation. The adversary system, with lay jurors as the usual ultimate factfinders in criminal prosecutions, has historically permitted triers of fact to draw on the standards of their community, guided always by limiting instructions on the law. To require a state to structure obscenity proceedings around evidence of a national community standard would be an exercise in futility.

Justice Douglas says in his dissent that the problem is that "One cannot say with certainty that material is obscene until at least five members of this Court, applying inevitably obscure standards, have pronounced it so. . .What shocks me may be sustenance for my neighbor. What causes one person to boil up in rage over one pamphlet or movie may reflect only his neurosis, not shared by others. . . .To send men to jail for violating standards they cannot understand, construe and apply is a monstrous thing to do in a nation dedicated to fair trials and due process." Nevertheless, Justice Douglas was in the minority and the philosophical hues of the Supreme Court will inevitably change from time to time leaving the question of relativism versus fixed standards in a continual state of flux. One might also expect that judges will be even less reluctant to let community standards control the question of what constitutes the practice of medicine than they might be in abandoning the question of obscenity to the jury. Judges will probably assume that everyone, both Defendants and jurors, knows what acts fit within the conventionally accepted definition of the practice of medicine.

THE METAPHYSICAL BACKGROUND TO TRADITIONAL HEALING IN NIGERIA

Chief K. O. K. Onyioha

To understand the practices of Traditional Healers in Nigeria, one needs to look a bit into some aspects of the metaphysics that support and sustain the people's traditional life. I am basing my statements on traditional healing among the Ibos, and on Ibo metaphysical concepts, for if a discussion must be pointed, it must pick on a guinea-pig from which inferences can be drawn to explain the behaviours of related communities.

The metaphysics of a people include the people's own theories about how the world began and their own concept of cosmology. These theories and concepts affect their ways of life, and so one can only appreciate the practices of Traditional Healers in Nigeria against the people's metaphysical concepts—which as a matter of fact, are the solid background against which Traditional Healers in Nigeria lean their practices.

The Ibos have their own theory about how the world began, who was the first man, and who was the first woman. To the Ibos, "Chineke," that is, "God the Creator," made everything in this world. He then created the first man and his name was Ife Nta. Ife in this name means Light, and Nta means "Small or Junior." And so the name of the first man in Ibo cosmology, interpreted in English means Junior Light. For this the Ibos call humanity—"Nde Ife," that is "Ife's Children." Some parts of Ibo land like Onitsha and Aro Ibos pronounce "Ndi Ife" as "Ndi Ive." Here "Ive" has some resemblance to the Jewish legend about Eve excepting that the sexes are juxtaposed. For while "Ive" in the Ibo legend is a man, Eve in the Jewish legend about the beginnings is a woman. The first woman in Ibo legend about the beginnings was called "Obuo-Omaranya" which means "Beauty in the Distance" and which is composite of the transient qualities of a woman. In the distance a woman shimmers resplendent beauty and is very attractive to a man. The man brings her into his house, she soon looses her shine and falls into her environment and the man looks outside again for another shimmering beauty in the distance. Tested against this, our experience of man to woman relationship in human society everywhere, this legend of ancient Ibos about Obuo Omara Anya (Beauty in the Distance) as name of the first woman created by Chineke (God the Creator) tends to look logical.

After Chineke (God the Creator) had created these first two humans—Ife Nta and Obuo-Oma-Ra-Anya—He, Chineke, sat them to a lecture on His Creations one day and said:

> "You are my Children. You cannot die. You have two-selves, metaphysical self which is your soul (Muo in Ibo) which is immortal like me; this is your real self which is one with me—it can never die. Your second self is the physical expression of your soul. This body can wither with age and time and collapse and allow your soul to assume a new physical frame to re-incarnate and continue its existence on earth. Everything I have created—the animals, including the lions, and the snakes, and all the plants, are "Nmamma" which means for your goodness and well-being. None is intended to harm you. If you mix them in their appropriate cosmic relationships the result will always be to enhance your happiness on earth. I will not show you all at once how to use them because if I do, you would want to finish all of them in one fell gulp, and these things would not last forever to perpetuate your existence on this earth which I have made your permanent home. Meanwhile, however, I give you only two fruits, Nkoro and Akpa—to live on till by experience, and trials and error, you will be able to find out for yourselves the values of these things and how to use them to enhance your welfare on earth. I will be with you always."

Then Chineke spoke to them in proverb: "I ge Nti Ali Ganu Ikiti Okpa Nanda" which means—if you listen very carefully to the ground you will hear the footsteps of ants— that is, if you listen inwardly to yourself, you will hear my faint voice within you telling you what to do on your hour of need and telling you what is right or wrong. This to the Ibos became the first proverb man learnt from Chineke.

The Ibo legend about creation said that it was at this first session with Chineke (God the Creator) that man's first spoken word was learned and it was Mmamma—and so when the Ibos gather to a meeting, the leader will begin by addressing the people saying: "Ndi Ibeanyi Mmamma ni—o!"— which is a short expression with very deep meaning:

"Brothers and Sisters: let every way of your lives be light; let all our acts be crowned with good." Evaluating this first philosophy of the Ibo, on the balance of logic, one sees something interesting in Chineke's presentation of Nkoro and Akpa to the first two humans as food that could sustain them till they found out the value of all the things of the world, because Nkoro and Akpa belong to the bean family of grains, full of protein and therefore capable of sustaining man without the need for eating meat. This first philosophy of the Ibo, though sounding naive and simple, has much influence on his thinking and attitudes to life. He believes that no man ever dies, believes in reincarnation because in his legend about the beginnings, Chineke told Ife Nta and Obuo-Omara-Anya that their souls are immortal, that they will reincarnate and the world is their permanent home. For this the Ibo believes that the soul of his ancestor is always hovering around, still playing his role as a father from his metaphysical existence to protect him against all metaphysical forces, and to influence his fortunes on earth. Because he believes in reincarnation, he holds that if you do good in your present life you will reincarnate in your next life to reap whatever you sowed. Thus, ancient Africans before the corrupting influences of foreign cultures, strove to do good to reap goodness in their reincarnation. And because Chineke, in his first talk to Ife Nta and Obuo Omaranya, had told them that everyone of his creations is for their own good and well being. The Ibos see beauty in the totality of being and identify man as symbolic of that beauty in life by calling man a symbolic name, Madu, which stretched out means Mma Di Na Ndu or Mma Ndu which means "there is beauty in life" or there is goodness in every way of life—or the beauty of life.

This first philosophy enjoined research where Chineke said to Ife Nta and Obuo Omaranya: "I will not tell you the uses of all my creations, you will have to find out these things for yourselves in course of time"—and compromises Ibo metaphysics with physical sciences. This is different from the Hebrew legend of the Bible in which God did not want Adam and Eve to know anything or to find out anything for themselves but chased them out of the Garden of Eden for eating the forbidden apple and becoming wise. Thus African metaphysics is not antagonistic to physical sciences of experimentation and conclusion, like European metaphysics of Aquinas, which for centuries set itself against physical sciences—treating it as heretic and through inquisitions killed and oppressed many scientists like Galileo who had tried to pry into the secrets of nature. From this portion of the legend it is clear that the Ibo's philosophical attitude is pragmatic and empiric and hardly superstitious and naive. He believes only what he has experienced. And most Black Africa is like that.

Because in his legend about creation, Chineke had told Ife Nta that all creations are for his goodness, that if he mixes them in their appropriate cosmic relationships he will obtain helpful results, and that even the lions, and the snakes are not intended to harm him, many communities of Eastern Nigeria live in harmony with large snakes. They don't kill snakes and snakes don't harm them. Thus the sanity of the Ibo legend that the lions could have been lying together in happy companionship with men if men had not turned hostile to them. History has it that a village in Owerri called Umuohiagu used to live in harmony with leopards till Christianity came and cut for them the cosmic cord that linked them in harmony with the leopards. The Ibos call leopard "Agu," and the name of the village, Umuohiagu in which the word "Agu" occurs is said to have derived from the fact that the people of this village of Eastern Nigeria used to live in harmony with leopards. The practices of traditional healers in Eastern Nigeria are very much influenced by this legend. Thus traditional healers sort a number of leaves and animals in their cosmic relationships and put them together to produce healing effects. No creature is valueless to traditional healers, not only in Eastern Nigeria but also in all Nigeria. The snails, snakes, skulls of dead humans, milipedes, centipedes, tortoise, lice, eggs, chickens, chalk, kola nuts and all manners of plants and animals are sorted together to produce curative effects.

Realising that some traditional healers used to incorporate snails in the treatment of certain ailments, Dr. Ayodele Tella of the Lagos University's Medical School, three years ago began a systematic in-depth investigation into the therapeutic potentials of the giant African snails. Dr. Tella came up with some interesting discoveries. He found out that when patients with excessive or moderate hypertension at the Lagos University Teaching Hospital were given daily rations of snails their blood pressure was considerably reduced. The result of Dr. Tella's research was published in screaming headlines in the Nigerian Daily Times of March, 1973 which read—"Good News for Victims of Hypertension: Snails Now Effective Remedy" The publication ended with an advice for all saying—"it will do you a lot of good to eat snails because you do not know whether that headache you have may be a sign of hypertension." The message which this story conveys to European medical science is that it can learn from Africa's traditional healings to enhance itself. For it goes without saying that there are cases in which Nigeria's traditional healers succeed where European medical science had failed. This is not to say that one is superior to the other; I am merely saying that none should denounce or despise the other, they should be complementary to each other, for obviously each has something new to lend to the other.

There are two kinds of traditional healers or native doctors in Nigeria. One is Dibia Nsi (Ibo) or the herbalist who may be said to be a physical scientist in the sense that he uses physical materials which get into physical contact with the patient he is treating. The other is Dibia Ogba Aja (Ibo) or the metaphysician. The Dibia Ogba (herbalist) may not be a seer. He merely knows herbs. The Dibia Ogba Aja is the seer versed in metaphysical sciences governed by his African traditional concept of cosmological hierarchy; but both the Dibia Nsi and the Dibia Ogba Aja work hand in hand in compromise of Africa's traditional physical science with traditional metaphysical science.

The Ibos in their cosmology hold that the Forces of Nature are departmentalized—with each Department headed by a spirit Force. In this cosmic hierachy they have Anyanwu, (sun) standing above all as declaring the overall powers of Chineke, God the Creator. There is no shrine dedicated to Anyanwu, and there is no priest exclusive to it. But all traditional healers, in making offerings to propitiate any spirit, first say, looking skywards, and holding his hands above his head: "Chineke (God the Creator) gozie aja nkea" (bless this offering) and adds, raising the cock or whatever he is offering to the sun, "Anyanwu kam' n'enye oke" (It is to the Sun I am giving a share). He says this three times before he calls the Spirit he wants to propitiate to take the offering.

Next to the Sun in the traditional healer's structure of metaphysical hierarchy is Ofor Na Ogu which is the Spirit of the head of the Department of Justice. It has a priest and a forest shrine dedicated to it. When an issue is disputed in a community, or if a man is accused of a crime which he is denying, he is taken before Ofor Na Ogu shrine, to swear that he did not commit the offence being alleged against him. Ofor Na Ogu operates on the conscience of man and represents Chineke's faint voice of right or wrong mentioned earlier in the Ibo first philosophy. It is a nagging spirit embedded in the mind of man and nags the conscience of the guilty one to instantaneous or subsequent death. Its celebration demands a dog, a big cock, kola nut and alligator pepper.

Next to Ofor Na Ogu is Agwu Nsi—a female spirit whose role is that of linkage between the metaphysical and the physical world. She interprets, like a good public relations officer, between the two worlds. All traditional healers particularly the Dibia Ogba Aja (Metaphysicians) are under her. She uses them to speak to mortal men. She conscripts individuals into her services. First, she descends upon and possesses the one she wants to make a native doctor or traditional healer. The individual begins to behave abnormally. All his affairs begin to go zig-zag. The chaos he experiences in his affairs compels him to consult a Dibia Ogba Aja or metaphysician, who divines and tells him—"Well, Agwunsi (Agwu Nsi) has taken possession of you. She wants you to serve her. Unless you follow her and get initiated into the society of native doctors, things will never again go well with you." Upon this explanation, the victim makes preparations, buys all the ingredients necessary for his initiation ceremony. Initiation of candidates into the society of traditional healers takes place only once a year. When the day comes, he is initiated, shown all the secrets of native doctors. Certain leaves are crushed and their water squeezed into his eyes to make him see double—to see both the spirits and men and to hear the messages of the spirit world and to see far into the future and make forecasts.

Originally native doctors became such only through possession or conscriptions by Agwu Nsi. Because of this, they wielded great influence in Ibo traditional society. Rich men longed to belong to their society and were willing to pay any charge for initiation—even though not chosen by the spirit head of the society—Agwu Nsi. Such "mechanical" native doctors were more often than not inefficient—they would not divine successfully, they would claim to cure everything but without curing anything. From this corruption of the group, native doctors or traditional healers began to lose their reputation and respect in Nigeria. People began to look down upon their practices because quacks had invaded their field and deceived people to collect money. Quacks charge heavily, whereas the real traditional healers who were conscripted into her services by the spirit Agwu Nsi would not charge much. They hold that they were given their healing powers to help their fellow man and not to amass wealth. They even believe that if they charge too much their powers would desert them. And so more often than not, the good traditional healers will say to you, after treating your case— "pay me anything you like." Sometimes they will treat you and say—"go and try my prescription first, if you succeed then come and pay me anthing you like."

Apart from this invasion by quacks, Christianity and European medical practitioners came up with denigration campaigns against traditional healers and their practices as superstitious, primitive, unhygienic and dangerous. The children of these traditional healers were attracted away from their fathers into schools for European system of Christian Education, and so they were no longer interested in understudying their fathers to learn the art of traditional healing and the secrets of their metaphysical practices.

In the cosmological hierarchy of the Ibos of Eastern Nigeria, Igwe or Kamalu or Amadi-Oha—the aliases reflect dialectical variations of the Ibos—is the spirit at the head of the sky with all the forces of nature like the rain, wind, lightning and thunder that emanate from the sky. So Igwe is popularly known as the Spirit of Thunder and Lightning. It is equivalent to Shango in Yoruba metaphysics or Ekpeinyong in Efik metaphysical hierarchy. It has a forest shrine and a priest devoted to it. It is propitiated in annual celebrations with ram or cock, palm wine, kola-nut and alligator pepper. It protects the community against secret or bad medicine which an enemy must have sneaked into the village. The people of eastern Nigeria believe that lightning never strikes anybody unless the person has committed a crime unknown to the people; and that it never strikes any place unless in the place is hidden something dangerous to the well being of the community. The Thunder Spirit has on many occasions in the people's experience been known to have defined the boundary of a disputed land, with a flash of lightning. So it became the practice of land disputants to go to the Priest of Igwe at its Forest Shrine to place their case. On that occasion they go with a ram, palm wine, kola nut and alligator pepper. In the experience of the people, claimants of the lands which did not belong to them had been badly shaken by lightning, or been carried off from their beds into the street during rains, or their houses smashed.

Ala is the spirit in charge of all lands of the people. It is the custodian of the people's moral traditions or laws of the land or code of ethics which the Ibos call Nso Ala or Omenani. For example, the traditional incest taboos. However, in our traditional context, family does not limit itself to the immediate nuclear group of father, mother and children, but involves the extended family system which embraces the 100th cousin. All these must not inter-marry unless the taboo is waived with permission from Ala. This may happen if by mistake the two relatives had mated and caused pregnancy which compels marriage. Ala has its forest shrine and its priest. Ala is most difficult to propitiate if offended by anybody violating the traditional code of ethics. The Ibos call such offence "Imeru Nso Ala" or Ime Ife Ala Naso Nso." It is most difficult to propitiate because of the very wide assortment of ingredients entailed. Ala spirit demands sheep, tortoise, flies, ant, beetle, feathers, chicken, hen, Abuke, Okuku Ayagheri, chameleon, dog, male and female lizards, snail, odo, chalk and of course Kola nut and alligator pepper. Because of the heavy toll Ala spirit takes, everybody wants to behave within the traditional code of ethics.

After Ala, comes Imo Miri Ochie, which is the Spirit responsible for all bodies of water in the world—streams, rivers, lakes and oceans. It has male and female. The male is called Imo Miri Ochie; the female is called Ekwuru Ochie. They are respectively equivalent to the merman and the mermaid in English. They are supposed to control childbirth. Couples in search of children, and girls who are about to get married go to the Imo Miri shrine usually situated by the waterside to make sacrifices. There is an annual festival called "Ezizza Iyi" dedicated to this spirit in many parts of Eastern Nigeria. The Ijaws call this Spirit "Owu," while the Efiks call it "Ndem." The people's philosophical or metaphysical concept around this spirit is the same all over Eastern Nigeria. While Imo Miri or Ndem is a water spirit, yet for areas without water there is a forest shrine dedicated to it. This spirit is believed to be capable of expressing itself in various forms as—python, beautiful maiden, crocodile, tortoise, or turtle, fish, etc. At its forest shrine in areas without water, one would always find tortoise and white snail. At its shrine at Adum-Ama, down Abonnema Way in the Rivers State hangs a huge old python with shimmering scales attended to by a white clad Adum Priest. People come from far and near to ask for any sort of favour excepting anything that would injure a man.

A woman wanting a child goes to her with sheep, cock, hen, lizard, long basket, eggs and black cloth. This spirit is believed to bring money. In the Rivers Areas, this spirit is the most powerful one among the peoples of the Niger Delta which is understandable because the people have more water than land, and the Spirit which commands such lion share of their territory should be the most powerful. Thus there is no facet of life in the Rivers Provinces of Eastern Nigeria which is not influenced by the Owu—art, culture, religion, marriage customs, aesthetics, morals, music and dances and masquerades.

Last, but not the least, is Fijoku or Ahiajoku or Njoku— the spirit responsible for all plants, and therefore the spirit in charge of agricultural undertakings. It is this that bestows wealth in our traditional society. A great annual festival—the New Yam Festival—is dedicated to it every year, in the same way as the Romans dedicated the festival of Saturnalia to Saturnus until Christians adopted it as Christmas celebration of the birthday of their Christ. Both festivals are alike in many respects: first, both festivals are in the wet season—the New Yam Festival is held in the rainy month of August in Nigeria; while the Saturnalia is held in the wintry month of December; secondly, both festivals are dedicated to the god of agriculture; and thirdly, both festivals mark for both the Nigerians and the Romans the end of a year and the beginning of a new one; and each of the festivals lasts for a week in the various months they are celebrated which is 7 days in Rome while our native week in our Nigerian tradition is 8 days. Thus it can be said that Nigeria has its own traditional equivalent of the Christmas which is the New Yam Festival, and with which the Godian Religion of Nigeria will untimately replace Christmas celebration in Nigeria.

In the above metaphysical system are seven spirits— namely, in descending order of magnitude—(1) Sun (2) Ofo Na Ogu, for justice (3) Agwunsi, for relations between the metaphysical and the physical worlds (4) Igwe, for the sky and its forces including rain, wind, lightning and thunder (5) Ala, for the land and its code of ethics (6) Imo Miri with Ekwuru Ochie, for all bodies of water (7) Fijoku for agriculture and wealth. Each of these spirits is not held by the Ibos as a god in its own right. Cosmos to them is a unity over which Chineke, God the Creator, is the supreme force and president while all the spirits are symbolic expressions or personifications of the various facets of his force necessary for psychological mobilisation in the metaphysical practices of traditional healers. So when a healer goes to the shrine of Igwe, for instance, he focuses his mind on invoking that particular aspect of Chineke's powers to serve his needs.

The traditional healers' metaphysics is not part of the people's religion. The religion of the people is usually headed by the Head Chief of the community who is both the spiritual and secular authority among his subjects. As a matter of fact, most parts of Ibo land, worship Chineke, God the Creator, only once in a year in two ceremonies spread over eight days. The Head Chief conducts the ceremonies called in Nkporo and Abiriba clans of Ohafia Division of Eastern Nigeria—Iwusi Oji which is the preliminary ceremony, and the Ogbo ceremony which is the main ceremony, which holds the people in religious unity. Unfortunately those who do not understand African religion declare to all the world that Africa is a pagan or an pan-theist culture even though monotheism came from Africa to humanity.

Hinduism is held as a civilised religion which compares with Christianity and Islam. Its metaphysics hold Brahman as supreme being or absolute spirit who works through a triad of—Brahma, the Creator of the universe, Vishnu, the preserver of the world; and Siva who represents both destruction and reproduction—just exactly in the same way as the traditional healers of Nigeria departmentalised the forces of Chineke, into seven departments under seven spirits. Thus I assume no reader would deride Nigeria's traditional healers as naive in their cosmological system.

It is important that every traditional healer of Ibo land understand this metaphysical structure if he is to render efficient services to his client. Obviously he must know which spirit is responsible for what, and which one he will propitiate over his client's problems. He must understand these forces of nature and how to bend them to his will. Consequently, good traditional healers do not divorce themselves from witchcraft, which is merely an attempt by man to bend the forces of nature to his will. Though some of those who have acquired the power of witchcraft have abused it in molesting their fellowman, yet the basic purpose of witchcraft is to serve the best interests of man. A good number of Nigeria's traditional healers acquire witchcraft to help them in their traditional healing—to help their clairvoyance and to keep others with witchcraft from obstructing their practices.

Let us recall then, that there are two classes of Traditional Healers in Eastern Nigeria—the Dibia Nsi who is the herbalist and the Dibia Ogba Aja, who is the metaphysician. The metaphysician is the seer and of him people say—"igakwu Oke Dibia Ogbakwu Oke Muo" which means

213

"if you run to a great traditional healer, he runs to a great spirit." So if a client comes to a traditional healer the first thing the native doctor does is to divine in order to ask the spirit Agwunsi, who I mentioned is the public relations officer of the metaphysical world, what is the cause of his client's trouble. Divination is the traditional healer's diagnostic method. The Ibos call it "Igba Aja" or "Igba Afa." Before he begins to divine, he first chews alligator pepper and spits at his shrine. This is to wake the spirit up or to call the spirit's attention to the presence of his client and his readiness to engage the spirit. After this he breaks kola nut, chews his bit, gives a share to his client, and throws some bits into his shrine for the spirit. The philosophy of kola in the metaphysical practices of the traditional healer is to get into covenant with the spirit and bind him to be honest to him in his dealings with him, because in the Ibo legend about kola nut, one is bound to be faithful to a man with whom one has eaten kola—you must not lie against him, you must not plan evil against him, you must not have anything to do with his wife, you are bound to protect and defend him. That is why kola is very important in Ibo traditional system of hospitality. A stranger comes into your house—you give him chalk paste on his wrist, and give him kola nut which he breaks and eats with you—you have by this simple act initiated him into the membership of your family with equal right of inheritance of property and title for the period he will stay with you. Thus the stranger immediately ceases to be regarded as such by the community. If he commits a crime and runs away, you are responsible. The chalk paste is symbolic of the clarity of heart or of the sincerity with which you have welcomed the stranger. So when the traditional healer offers kola to the spirit at his shrine, he binds the spirit to serve his needs.

After kola nut, he offers chalk to the spirit and to his client as a declaration of sincerity in the transaction between him, the spirit and his client. Then he offers yellow Odo wood to the spirit, and his client, as symbolic of peace which will govern their coming together in the consultation. After these preliminary offerings of kola, chalk, odo and alligator pepper, the traditional healer begins his divination diagnostic exercises, He casts his "Afa" which are special seeds, or cowries, or pieces of kola nut, for divination, and reads it; casts and re-casts them till the spirit Agwu Nsi tells him through the Afa what has caused the ailment and what treatment should be applied. This divination is a metaphysical science which only the traditional healers study and understand. It involves numerology, and depends also on the cadence of the "Afa", whether it falls face up or face down when it is cast. As he casts the Afa, he may be drumming, singing, saying in-cantations and calling on the public relations spirit Agwunsi, and the names of his ancestors from whom he inherited the practice. They may divine and tell the client—"Well, your trouble is caused by Figioku (the spirit of agriculture) because you went to your neighbor's farm and uprooted his crops." He then prescribes the materials which the client will use to propitiate the spirit in order to regain his health. He does that and gets well without actually drinking any medicine into his system. Or he may divine and tell his patient that witch-craft is the cause or that his enemy had poisoned him, or that the spirit of his dead father is worrying him because he had not performed all the necessary burial ceremonies. In each case he prescribes ingredients necessary for the sacrifices to ward off the evil influences. The traditional healer may divine and say,—"well, what is wrong with you is simply biological—there are no metaphysical forces involved." In this case he may direct the patient to a traditional healer who is a Dibia Nsi or Herbalist, for the appropriate herbal treatment for his illness. Sometimes the metaphysician may apply the herbs himself.

Traditional healers don't diagnose diseases by palpating or fingering the body of the patient like European medical doctors do, who strip naked the patient and finger about the private parts of any woman who comes to them for maternity treatment. They diagnose by metaphysical means. In fact, some of the very good traditional healers have acquired such clairvoyance that you come into their shrine, they tell you all your problems before you make your complaints. This sounds stranger than fiction, but it is as true as any truth can be.

History is philosophy teaching by examples and I con-sider it would be a dramatic illustration to you of the powers of Nigerian traditional healers if I narrate some of my personal experiences with traditional healers. Before these experiences, I simply had no regard for them because of the Christian system of education through which I was brought up from childhood—Christian system of education which made it its duty to brainwash all African children to hate everything African.

On May 12, 1952, my wife, Mrs. Ngozi Onyioha, who was pregnant with my second daughter went to a Government Maternity Hospital in Lagos—the Massey Street Dispensary, for examination. The Gynecologist of the Maternity Hospital examined her, and reported the position of the child as lying across the stomach. The gynecologist was then, as he is now, my personal friend. She was informed that unless the child changed position, delivery would be difficult and surgery might be necessary. At that date my wife was only eight days from delivery. The medical personnel could not see the chance of the child turning right within the next seven days. However, they decided to tie a band of cloth round her stomach as a means of forcing the child to turn. That band of cloth around her stomach made the already suffocating pregnant woman very uncomfortable. On the following day, May 13, 1952, we carried the complaint to a traditional healer at Ajegunle, Apapa, and told him how worried we were that my wife was due for delivery in seven days—about May 20, 1952—while the child was still lying high across the stomach. We told him we feared the possibility of surgery. The traditional healer smiled and told us that my wife would not need an operation. As we sat with him in his consulting room, he picked up a piece of native chalk from his shrine. He called his daughter to bring a cup of water, and sent my wife to buy for him one ripe banana and a white plate. He ground the native chalk and put it into the plate. He then peeled the ripe banana and cut it into seven slices representing the number of days remaining for my wife to be due for delivery. As he was mixing the ingredients—chalk, banana and water in the white plate, he murmured some incantations —for traditional healers use also the power of words. He then handed the plate to my wife with this direction for use— "Every morning, first thing before you take your breakfast, pick one piece of this ripe banana from the plate and eat. Do that daily at the rate of one piece of the ripe banana per day, for seven days. By the time you finish picking up the pieces of banana, your child will have turned and engaged properly for delivery, and you will deliver—no palaver." I was at that time Associate Editor of a leading newspaper in Nigeria—the West African Pilot. I had no faith in what he had given. I went simply for the psychological satisfaction that I was doing my best for my worried wife, for if I did not run around she would accuse me of not being interested in her problem. We came home with the parcel. Doubts criss-crossed in me as I could not see how mere water, ordinary chalk and banana, could turn a child in the womb when the hospital physicians could not do anything about it. The traditional healer had not asked me to pay a mite, he had merely asked my wife to go back to the maternity hospital after seven days for examination and return to report to him.

Exactly seven days after my wife had eaten the last bit of the banana in the morning, she began to feel some labour at 6 p.m. on the evening of May 20, 1952. I rushed her to the Massey Street Dispensary. Quickly the doctor was called in by the mid-wives on duty because they had known the case to be a problematic one. The doctor examined her and to his great surprise saw the child engaged and ready to come out. By 11 p.m., May 20, 1952, the child was born normally—my second daughter. In overflowing joy that no one had to rip my wife's stomach open I called the baby, Ngozi, which means Blessing. I told the traditional healer on May 21, 1952 that the child was delivered without trouble and he said—"I expected that." I bought beer to celebrate with him and then gave him money in gratitude.

This was my first experience with a traditional healer. My second experience was when the wife of a friend of mine had a very serious belly-ache in 1952. The senior brother of this friend was and still is a Canadian trained Medical Doctor. My friend carried the wife to his senior borther's clinic where she was given all sorts of treatment, but the belly-ache would not subside. For three days, the Medical Doctor battled with the belly-ache of his brother's wife without success. Then I suggested to my friend—"let's try that man who helped

217

my wife. They call him Baba Olodi." We went to his compound and he shouted—"Ah! my friend, you came again,
what's the matter?" We told the story while my friend's
wife writhed with stomach pain on the floor.

We naturally expected the native doctor would squeeze
some powerful herbs into the cup for her to drink. But no,
Baba Olodi asked us to carry the woman into his shrine—a
white washed small house. Then he locked the woman up in
the shrine and came out. He called all his children, dressed
all of them in white cloth, and then picked up his native
harp and started playing and singing and dancing with the
children. My friend and I were not enjoying what we considered a huge joke. Here we are with a woman who has been
crying for the past three days with stomach pain and you
think this is the right time for you to start dancing with your
children instead of finding some medicine for her to drink.
He did not care about our reaction—he danced on, sang on,
and played his harp with his children. After about an hour,
we heard some knocks at the locked door of the shrine—it
was my friend's wife knocking from inside. We thought the
woman was fed up with Baba Olodi's neglect. The native
doctor stopped the dancing, walked up to the shrine and
opened the door. To our surprise, instead of a raving, crying
woman, we saw my friend's wife in broad smiles—the pains
had gone! She was alright, she said. With thanks not unmixed
with fear, we gave Baba Olodi what money we had. Stranger
than fiction, but yet true. This is just one of the wonders of
some of our traditional healers in Nigeria—curing without
physical contact—curing with drumming, songs, and dances—
curing by witchcraft!

Here is another "case history," from the same healer. In
1949 I married. On December 3, 1950 I had my first child, a
girl. As you know, a man always wants his first child to be a
boy. Thus I was not quite pleased, but friends consoled me
with the fairy tale that to have a girl as first child is good luck.
Then I am a lucky man, I mused, and took heart. The next
pregnancy came and the child was born on May 20, 1952—
another girl. Ah, that was too much luck for me now. I refused to see my wife in the Maternity Hospital. But my
mother-in-law dragged me there. The third pregnancy came—

and another girl was born on August 27, 1953, and I nearly swooned. What could not be helped must be endured.

Worried, I went to the same native doctor, Baba Olodi, who had become my friend and lamented my problem of having female children. He brought out his working tools and began to divine into the situation. He looked up and told me—"Well K.O.K. your trouble is caused by the spirit of your dead father. He wants to reincarnate as the first son in your family so that he would be your successor and boss of the house. But he does not want to be born abroad, he wants to be born in your village. So he is waiting for you to come home before he reincarnates. While you are here in Lagos he will not come, nor will he allow any other male child to be born in your house. And so if you must have a male child in the next pregnancy of your wife, you've got to go home."

On December 23, 1953, I gathered my wife and things from Lagos and returned home—to Nkopro in Eastern Nigeria—arriving December 24, 1953. In 1954 my wife became pregnant in the village. In the second month of the pregnancy, my wife had a dream in which she heard a great noise of jubilation in the village square—everybody was shouting—"Onu Kama Bianwa" which means "Onu Kama is coming." Still in the dream, she looked out into the village square—through our bedroom window. She saw my father coming. My wife did not know my father, but the description she made of the man in the dream was the exact picture of my father and the clothing he used to wear when he lived. He gave her a rafia purse to keep under her bed. My father was a produce buyer when he was alive and he used to go about his trade with the sort of rafia purse he was holding in the dream when my wife saw him. At first my wife did not keep the purse exactly where the dream-man wanted it to be kept. He shook his head, retrieved the purse, and again told her where he wanted the bag kept. She put it in the right place, the dream-man nodded approval, and gave her a sign that he would be coming back later. Then he floated away to the gable end of our house. My wife woke in fright—heart beating wildly and sweating. She ran away from our bedroom to my uncle to whom she told the dream. I was not at home when this happened—I was 36 miles away at a Divisional

Council meeting in which I was the elected representative of the clan. When I returned she told me the story and added—"if I have a boy by this pregnancy it must be your father."

When my wife was due to deliver, I took her to a maternity home in Umuahia. At the Maternity Home on May 20, 1955 she delivered a baby—her first baby boy! But to my wife's dismay, the boy would not cry, and would not open its eyes. The midwife did everything to induce the baby to cry and to open its eyes, but it would not. My wife began to cry. She thought the child was abnormal. Everybody was embarrassed and a messenger was sent to call me from the Council meeting. The messenger did not tell me what anxiety was going on at the maternity over the child—he simply came and told me that my wife had delivered. What did she deliver, I asked, and he said—a boy. I cut capers and double paced. I had long made up my mind that I would call him my father's name and so as soon as I got to the maternity home and I was led into the labor room where the baby was still lying because he had not yet cried, I called the child by my father's name—Onu Kama. Then he emitted a shrill cry, opened his eyes and blinked at me three times and closed them. Everyone was surprised. They told me the story and I said—"Well, maybe the old man wanted me as his son to be first man on earth he would see and talk to at his reincarnation." In this drama was a fulfillment on March 20, 1955, of the clairvoyance of a native doctor, Baba Olodi of Ajegunle, Apapa, Lagos, an Urhobo man, which was made in 1953.

Am I by these short stories giving you an insight into how traditional healers operate in Nigeria? After all, knowledge derives from the experiences of individuals retold. The tragedy is that this Urhobo healer died in 1962.

Let us look at another case. I was eager to have male children and because of that I was not giving my wife any breathing space. Within four years and nine months—December 3, 1950 and March 20, 1955—we had four children. After my first son came in 1955 I expected the floodgate for males had opened. But the child that followed was a girl, and the next was another girl—that gave me five girls and one boy. But after the last girl born March 21, 1958, difficulties arose. Each time my wife missed her period, the last female child would scream in the middle of the night, my wife would jump up from her sleep, scream, and at once start to bleed—abortion. This happened with every pregnancy. We consulted a gynaecologist at the Government Hospital in Umuahia, Eastern Nigeria. He was trained in England and had a great reputation and still does. He examined her, subjected her to all sorts of treatments—D & C operation, and a series of injections. But every time my wife missed her period, the girl would scream in the middle of the night and my wife would wake up with another abortion. For nearly two years this continued to our chagrin while the hospital had nothing more to do for us. Since I had left Lagos and Baba Olodi behind, I knew of no good traditional healer I could rely on to treat my case in Eastern Nigeria. One day my wife's aunt suggested we should see a traditional healer called Moses in Nkata Na Ugba village of Umuahia Ibeku in Eastern Nigeria. I took my wife there—expecting no salvation, but just to satisfy my sister-in-law.

At his consulting room—which is his Shrine,—we told him my wife's troubles. We told him we had one wicked child who did not want to see another child born in our family. After listening to our story, the Native Doctor drew close to his shrine, picked up his tortoise shell and began to knock discordant notes on it. As he knocked, he called the names of his ancestors who had handed the practice to him, inviting them to come to his aid in solving the problem. Then, he broke kola nut, alligator pepper, offered chalk and yellow wood, and then began his divination for diagnosis. As he played with his "Okwo" he was singing weird songs, mumbling some words calling on Agwu Nsi, the Public Relations Spirit—all in Ibo. Then he looked up and said:— "K.O.K., that child you call a wicked child is in fact the saviour of your wife. Your wife's uncle, called Chinyerem Nwaogboso, died two years ago. While he lived he loved your wife very much. He wants to take your wife to live with him in the spirit world. He wants to take her through pregnancy. The man who had been coming and for whom your wife has been missing her period has been the uncle with the sinister intention—pretending to be reincarnating through your wife only to kill her during labour. The little daughter you now call wicked, being herself still very close to the spirit world is able to see through the wicked intention of your uncle, and so screams to frighten him away each time she sees him coming into your womb after you have missed your period. So you should thank this child for keeping you alive. Now, I tell you what to do. Buy a white sheep with no black spot, buy two yards of white shirting, a hen, two yards of black shirting. In the middle of the night, take these things to a disused road. Wrap the sheep with these cloths in the way dead bodies are wrapped, and bury it alive in the middle of the disused road. Leave the hen to wander away in any direction it cares. By this exercise you have exchanged your wife with the sheep in the wicked plan of the spirit and trapped your uncle himself to live when he comes into your womb. After you have done this, and your daughter screams again and you have another abortion, come and report to me, and I will burn down my shrine for letting me down."

I was not satisfied with this. I told him: "Look Moses, I have not come to play. Look for some medicine—gather some herbs—give my wife medicine." He replied: "Well, K.O.K., Agwocha dilam, I have finished my prescription and my treatment."

Reluctantly, I left with my wife. He did not ask for a penny and I gave him nothing because I did not believe him. However, just to please my wife, I went places and bought all the things and buried them in the middle of the night, as he had directed. When my wife again missed her period, our little girl did not scream again, and the baby was delivered at Port Harcourt on July 4, 1960—a boy. But seven days after the child was delivered, he developed a high fever. Nothing our family doctor in Port Harcourt General Hospital did could bring the fever down. My wife herself became very sick with fever too and I began to run around again. When nothing worked, I remembered to take them to Moses in Umuahia. When we arrived at his compound, I tolk him the story of the child's fever and that of the mother too. He laughed, and turned to the child and said—"Enyi, onye biara nga nwanne ya omere ife ojo tusianu"—which means: "My friend, has a person who comes to his sister's house done any harm? Cool off now." Then he turned to us and said—"That's your uncle I told you about. He only wants to have his identity declared for all to know that he has reincarnated." Then he held the child by the hand and called him by the name of the dead uncle. And he said to him—"Now that we have declared your identity we expect you will now cool down."

He told us to buy a cock, send it to the oldest man of the compound where the uncle had lived, and ask him to cook the cock and call everybody in the compound to come and eat and to declare to the gathering while they ate the cock that Nwaogboso had reincarnated. He told us not to take the child to the compound where the feast would be held. He said there was no need for any medicine when I asked for medicine for both of them. What he had directed should be done was all they needed. On our way back to Port Harcourt, we bought a cock and sent it to the late uncle's compound. By the time we reached Port Harcourt, forty miles away, the fever had come down for both the child and the mother. Stranger than fiction, yet so true.

Let us look at this other example. In January 1963, my wife was two months pregnant with our ninth baby, when we went home to Nkporo on leave from my job as Public Relations Manager of the Government-owned Eastern Nigeria Development Corporation. At about 10 p.m. one evening, my wife began to abort. I put her into our car and drove to Abiriba Joint Hospital—six miles away. At the hospital the doctor had gone to town and could not be easily located. We could not wait, with the bleeding increasing. We drove off to another hospital—Umunna Ato Hospital—sixteen miles away. That was already after 11 p.m., and the doctor had gone to bed. I woke him and told him our problem. He agreed to give my wife an injection to stop the bleeding but insisted that my wife must be admitted to the hospital after the injection. I told the doctor that I should be allowed to take my wife home after the injection, that we had enough comfortable home for a perfect rest, and that it would be too much of a trouble for me driving 16 miles thrice daily to give her the kind of food she would want to eat. The doctor would not yield. At this I decided to go and try my old friend Moses, the traditional healer of Umuahia—Ibeku, 36 miles away from my home. That was already about 12 midnight—the bleeding was increasing. By the time I reached his house at about 1 a.m. the traditional healer was fast asleep. I woke him and told him our problem. We were all standing in the open in his compound. Then he spoke to the spirits of his shrine saying: "My people, Onyioha and his wife have come. If your visit to a place was good, you repeat the visit. Now they have come again, and it is their wish that the wife's pregnancy does not abort." After saying this he went behind the shrine to a small palm tree and tore out one palm frond. He came to my wife—and placed the palm frond on her belly immediately above her navel and tied it up in a sort of noose. He handed the palm frond noose to me and said—"It's all over."

"What is over?" I asked. "Your wife won't bleed again," he said. "Look, Moses," I said, "I have not come here to joke, I came that you may give her medicine to drink to stop the bleeding." He replied: "I am through with it, she needs nothing more to drink. I bet that if the bleeding has not stopped before you reach home, I will burn up my shrine for letting me down if you bring back such a report to me." When I insisted that I wanted some medicine, he went again behind his shrine, collected some leaves and said: "When you reach home, first thing in the morning boil this with yam, crayfish, and fish, salt and pepper but no oil—and eat it with your wife for breakfast." Surprised, I asked him, "Why do I need to eat it with my wife, am I bleeding?" And he retorted: "Don't you want something to eat? It is now all over—It's now all over—good night." But before he went in he warned me: Don't allow that noose to get loose prematurely, for if it does your wife will deliver prematurely; don't allow it to get misplaced, for if you do your wife cannot deliver that baby and she must die. But when she is due to deliver you undo the noose and she will deliver safely. So you see, the life of your wife is in your hands to keep or lose." That was frightening enough. At once I handed the noose over to my wife—keep your own life. You can imagine her fright.

Back to our car we drove off on a return journey to our home 36 miles away. But by the time we reached Umunna Ato Hospital exactly nineteen miles away from the shrine of

Moses, my wife told me she felt no more bleeding. When we reached home, she examined herself and reported that she felt as if she never bled at all. We then came face to face with the problem of where to keep the miraculous noose for the whole period of pregnancy. We thought of the possibility of rats and cockroaches eating it, we thought of our rascally children picking it up and throwing it away. Where on earth must this thing be hidden away from danger for the balance of seven months pregnancy. A headache indeed! Then it occured to us, and we decided to put it at the bottom of my wife's box. We removed all her clothings, put the noose in its bare bottom; then spread layers of newspapers on it and packed back all of the clothing upon it. We thought we had done the job.

The pregnancy developed, and on July 14, 1963 when my wife began to have her labor pains, we dug out the noose and undid it, then rushed her to Park Lane Nursing Home, Enugu, where she had normal delivery of another baby boy—Chukwuemeka Onyioha. The boy's name means "God has done very well."

Africa's traditional healers, when you meet the true ones, are miraculous healers, and they are most marvelous in gynecology. If you doubt my story, follow me to Umuahia, bringing along with you a woman with problems. I will take you to Moses. He did it for me, he did it for the wife of a friend who had bled for three weeks even though under the treatment of Government hospital gynecologists at Enugu General Hospital; and he had been doing it for many more before I met him.

If a woman always aborts, just take her to Moses. He will simply tie a little string around her waist and the pregnancy will develop no matter whatever the strain or excitement to which you may subject the woman.

It will be no question of injection, no oral administration, but just a simple string around a woman's waist that does the trick. There are many traditional healers like Moses, each has his own style of the miracle. If you doubt me, follow me to Umuahia and I will take you to him.

In orthopedic medicine, Nigerian traditional healers are fantastic. European doctors soon get fed up with fractures and talk of amputation, while traditional healers in Nigeria take from hospitals cases readied for amputation, and treat them successfully. To prove this come with me to Enugu, and I will take you to a celebrated bone mender of Ngwo called Enwu Nweke. He has a wonderful X-ray style. His X-ray instruments comprise a rib of buffalo, and a staff of office in the form of a spear round which all manners of things are tied in two places—top and centre. The two instruments are very old and inherited through past generations of bone menders in the family. He calls the spear-like instrument "Oji." When a patient is brought to him and he wants to determine whether the problem is sprain, simple fracture or compound fracture, he sticks the spearlike instrument—the Oji—into the ground. He then touches the patient's broken part with the rib bone of the buffalo which the family's bone menders have been using from generation to generation, and touches the spear-like instrument with the bone also. By this contact he establishes invisible links between the broken part of the patient with his "Oji" spearlike "X-ray" instrument. He then holds the "Oji" with his left hand and watches the veins of his hand. As a visitor to his clinic, he invites you to watch his hand with him. Soon you see the middle vein of his hand rise under the skin and begin to move like a big worm up and down his hand. If he feels no bite of the worm-like vein, that lack of bite concludes for him that the problem is ordinary sprain; if he feels a slight bite, then it is a simple fracture; if the bite is serious, then compound fracture is the conclusion, and he proceeds to treat the patient accordingly. He has never been known to fail. Bone mending is the family's tradition. In orthopedic medicine the world has much to learn from Africa.

Traditional healers in Nigeria are indeed marvelous. Their methods of healing incorporate the physical science of the herbs of Dibia Nsi. Quite recently the traditional healer's chewing stick called "Kpako," commonly used in Nigeria, was found to contain properties which can revert a sickle cell to normal, by a hematologist of Ibadan University Teaching Hospital. This was given wide publicity in the Nigerian Daily Times between September and October, 1972 under a screaming headline—"New Hope for Patients of

Sickle Cell Anaemia."

Hypertension and sickle cell anaemia are ailments which hitherto have defied European medical science. But today from the giant African snail and the chewing stick used by the traditional healers of Nigeria, we are about to celebrate victory over these chronic diseases.

The healing method of traditional healers in Nigeria incorporates metaphysical sciences which include witchcraft—and the phenomena by which they affect their patients and effect a cure are intangible, invisible and therefore difficult to connect, describe and defend. I have been able to discuss this subject with confidence because I am speaking from personal experience. The tragedy of the metaphysical powers of traditional healers in Nigeria is that the results they produce are most of the time doubted and dismissed even by those who have benefited from them, as sheer coincidence. This is because Christianity in Africa has for many years devoted itself to the job of frightening people away from it as the devil's practice, superstitious, unreal and unwanted. But I know I have enough cultivation and sophistication to be able to determine what is real and what is coincidence and I don't see how any person can prove the experiences I have described as sheer coincidence. I do not think that Homer had seen as much of the wonders of traditional healers of Africa as I have already seen in my fifty years of life, before he wrote in the Odyssey that "in Africa the men are more skilled in medicine than any of human kind."

If one would go by what we are now seeing of hospitals in Nigeria one would be inclined to believe that European medical science is reaching to the end of its tether, and needs now to call off its professional jealousy, and investigate and learn what traditional healers are doing. There are many cases given up by hospitals as incurable which traditional healers have cured.

Another instance. In 1955, my wife was struck down after delivering my first baby boy by what the Medical Officer of Umuahia Government Hospital diagnosed as acute Anaemia. That kept my wife in a hospital bed for four months during which time she was subjected to blood transfusions and tablets like liver extract, folic acid, fersolate, multivite and so on, as the doctor prescribed. I bought all the prescriptions. None worked. It reached a stage when her heart began to stop beating regularly every Monday, Wednesday and Friday. And each time she was revived with an intra-veinous injection of nikethamide which the doctor advised that I should always make available. That became very expensive. He called me one day into his office and said: "K.O.K., I am very sorry about this, but I have to inform you that it does not seem that your wife is likely to survive this sickness. I think she will die. I would ask you to make arrangements to carry her away from the hospital." My wife discharged to death!

I went home with her and roamed the streets of Umuahia in despair, asking anyone I met—"please tell me, where can I get a native doctor to cure my wife." Many called a name, and I tried all, quacks and good ones alike. Each charged, and I paid. All I wanted was the life of my wife. The crowd I gathered the first day was useless but I had spent 27 pounds ($81.00) on them. It was on the following day that a friend of mine, Mr. Jumbo, directed me to go and see an Owerri woman called Mama Lucy. I went to her house. She would not allow me to tell her why I came because she said she knew. She asked me to give her two pounds ($6.00) and I did. She told me to go—that she would come.

For two days I did not see the woman. But one Friday, about 12 noon—I was not at home—this woman ran to my house, and commanded my bed-ridden wife to follow her— a woman who had lost all her hair and whose feet and palms had withered flat and yellow from bloodlessness—a woman who for all these months was stooling and urinating into bed pans—that was the woman this native doctor commanded to rise up and walk after her to her house!

My wife hesitated and then managed to get up and follow. Up a little hill of our street, they both went slowly until they reached her house. She put my wife into bed.

When I returned to my house I was frightened to see my wife gone. My servants told me that Mama Lucy came and took her away. How, by car or what, I asked. And the astonishing answer was that they both walked together. I ran to Mama Lucy's house where I saw my wife in bed. On seeing me the witch smiled and said: "A witch has plucked the heart of your wife and hung it on a tree. I had interferred against her harming your wife. It was fixed that the case could be tried at a meeting of the town's witches and wizards this Friday night, but the witch decided to kill her before the meeting tonight. That is why I rushed to come and take your wife to my own house. Let me see who will come and kill her in my house. You see, if I did not do that your wife would have died this afternoon."

I was silent. After some time, I left her. The following morning which was Saturday, I came to the woman to see my wife. The witch again told me—"You are lucky. Your wife will not die, the meeting of the witches did not find her guilty, and set her free." I thanked her with mixed feelings— more full of doubt than belief. The following morning which was Sunday, I came to Mama Lucy's house to see my wife. To my surprise, she was sitting up. She smiled, showed me her fingers and feet which until the previous day were simply flat and bloodless, now turgid with red blood! I turned to Mama Lucy with a look of awe, and she said—"Yes, you people give injections with needle. I have given her our own kind of injection. Last night I went out, sucked blood from people and sucked into her. What you need to do now is to take her to the hospital to give her injections to purify the blood I have sucked into her."

Here is a practical proof—I have seen my wife's flat fingers and feet full of red blood. Hurrah! My wife is born again, my wife will live. When she said: "Tomorrow, Monday, at 4 p.m. I will discharge your wife, but after a mock burial ceremony of her. By this ceremony she will be exchanged with the dead to appease those who wanted to kill her. So when you come on Monday, buy a mat, and two yards of white shirting and two yards of cloth called jioji." At the appointed time, I took all the things to her. She put the mat on the floor, and told my wife to lie on it face up—hands and legs completely stretched out. Then she turned to me and said: "I will spread these cloths over her like the head is laid in state." She picked up a piece of bark of wood called "Enunu Ebe" from her shrine and said: "The moment I place this bark on her breast she will become unconscious. She cannot hear again what we are saying. I will call her four times. At the fourth call they will release her with a forceful push from the Spirit world back to you. She will come straight on her heels and knees not bent at all. It will be your duty to catch her because if she falls she will be dead forever. Now it is up to you to catch your wife back from the spirit world alive."

The ceremony began, I took my position in front of my wife in such a way that she must fall straight into my arms when she is pushed. I spread out my arms—and swore: "now that it has all boiled down to a wrestle to keep my wife alive, my father was a great wrestler, I won't let them beat me—my wife must not drop from me—I must catch her alive."

Mama Lucy then placed the "Enunu Ebe" on my wife's breast and began the calls: (1) Ngozi Onyioha (silence), (2) Ngozi Onyioha (no answer), (3) Ngozie Onyioha (no answer), (4) Ngozi Onyioha—and up came my wife with force—you could feel she was actually pushed by an unseen hand—and straight into my spread arms she fell, I nearly fell with her, but no, it must not happen. I absorbed the shock and stood firm. Then I quietly lowered her into bed. She was unconscious, and I sat by her to wait for her to come round. After sometime she opened her eyes, smiled at me, and Mama Lucy said: "Now your wife is discharged."

Till today I have continued to pull the legs of the doctor who told me in 1955 that my wife would die. The lesson which this experience conveys is that physical science should now work together with metaphysical science to elongate the existence of man on this earth in a new civilisation in which neither would despise the other. If only one field of learning can agree that there is value in the other field worth investigating, if only every nation or race can accept that every other nation or race has something new also to teach humanity, we would have the secrets of the forces of nature around us for a richer, healthier and happier life.

TRADITIONAL MEDICAL PRACTICE AND THERAPEUTICS IN NIGERIA

A. Akisanya, Ph.D.

I would like to discuss in this essay traditional medicine and medical therapeutics with a view to highlighting some of the salient characteristics which convincingly demonstrate the ingenuity of the traditional doctors, and the dexterity of their practice. All these doctors without exception tried to diagnose ailments and were able to relate certain symptoms to specific diseases. Some even made a close study of dietary requirements of ailing patients, and were of the opinion that certain diseases, in order to be effectively cured demanded avoidance of certain types of food by the patient. All these are no more than extensions of the uses of natural resources which were fully exploited by these traditional doctors for the benefit of the human race.

The bible contains very little information on the subject of medical practices of old Testament times. The Garden of Eden contained all the natural vegetation which Adam and Eve ever needed for food and for medical care. However, there is abundant evidence from the factual account in the same old Testament of the high premium placed on social and personal hygiene by the people of that era. The Jews indeed are the greatest pioneers in public health.

The New Testament contains numerous vivid accounts of effective curative treatment of ailing patients by our Lord Jesus Christ. There was the case of the blind man whom Jesus treated by making a clay with His spittle, which He used to annoint the blind eyes. The blind man was then asked to go and wash the annointed eyes in the pool of Siloam, and his sight was restored. What about the story of the healing of the ten lepers; the woman with the issue of blood (now known as cancer of the womb); the restoration of life to the dying centurion servant, and to the daughter of Jairus? to mention quite a few of the patients whom Jesus treated and restored to normal health, making use of the traditional methods of prayer and faith in the power of God, the greatest Physician!

The early Greek physician, Erasitratus held that the chief cause of disease is excess of blood which he referred to as 'PLETHORA.' He was of the opinion that most plethoric diseases could be treated by diminishing the supply of blood to the diseased part by starvation. This reduction in supply of blood could be achieved by blood-letting, and it was the method much used by the contemporaries of Erasistratus. Erasistratus seldom employed this practice of blood-letting, and so his followers abandoned it. He was very much opposed to violent remedies, and the therapeutic methods which he adopted were exercise, vapour bath, and dietary control.

Traditional doctors from India were very good in the treatment of snake bites. According to history, Dhanvantari, a legendary figure, was deified as a god of medicine. But in later times, his status was gradually reduced until he was credited with having been an early king who died of snake bite. The story went on to recall the relations of Dhanvantari with snakes, and the skill with which early Indian traditional doctors treated snake bites. Some of the traditional doctors made use of magical methods in the treatment of diseases, and also charms in the expulsion of demons which traditionally were supposed to be the cause of diseases in ailing patients.

The Indian traditional doctors did classify disease, and used all the five senses in diagnosis. For instance, the sense of hearing was used to distinguish the nature of the breathing; alteration in voice, and the grinding sound produced by the rubbing together of the broken ends of bones. The therapeutics of the Indian physicians were mainly dietetic and medicinal. Dietetic treatment and dietary control were considered very important, and this took precedence over medical treatment. The most important methods of active treatment were known as the "FIVE PROCEDURES," and these consisted of: emetics, purgatives, water enemas, oil enemas, and sneezing powders. Inhalations were frequently prescribed, and very often, leeching, cupping and bleeding were employed in treatment as and when necessary.

The Indian traditional doctors placed great importance on personal hygiene and diet as requisites for effective curative treatment. This of course was a reflection of their very strict religious beliefs. Hygienic measures were prescribed, and fats were much used, both internally and externally. Not more than two meals a day were allowed the patients, and the nature of the diet including the condiments, was clearly indicated. The amount of water to be taken by the patient before and after meals was specified. The patient was required to bathe the body and to clean the teeth with extractives of particular herbs, and special oils from plants were prescribed for use as cosmetics.

Surgery was also practised by the Indian traditional doctors. Operations carried out included excission of tumors, incission of abscesses; punctures of collection of fluid in the abdomen; extraction of foreign bodies; expression of the contents of abscesses; probing of fistuls, and stitching of wounds. These doctors were outstanding in abdominal operations, particularly, the removal of stones in the bladder. Plastic surgery was also their speciality, and records show that adulterous citizens in those days, had their nose amputated as a punishment; the repair was then effected by cutting a piece of the required size and shape, from the cheek of the guilty person, which was then applied to the stump of the nose. In all these surgical operations, use was made of alcohol as a narcotic to reduce the pain of the patient. The instruments used were predominantly of steel, and included scissors, saws, needles, forceps, tubes, probes, hooks, and levers.

The Chinese Materia Medica consists of vegetable, animal (including human) and mineral remedies. Drugs like castor oil, camphor, cannabis sativa (Indian hemp), chaulmoogra oil (remedy for leprosy), ma haung—Ephedra vulgaris (which contains ephedrine) were introduced and used by the Chinese traditional doctors, long before the advent of the Western trained doctors and western medicine. The prescription for leprosy treatment is now being used by the western physicians, and ephedrine finds useful application in the hands of western physicians for the treatment of asthma. Immunisation technique was also known and employed by the Chinese physicians. This was practised in China in ancient times especially in the control of small pox by innoculation of the small-pox matter in order to produce a mild but immunising attack of the patient by the disease.

This technique was adopted in Europe in 1720, and has been in use since then till today all over the world.

It would perhaps be pertient at this stage to discuss briefly the basis of Chinese traditional medicine. Chinese traditional doctors founded their practice on the dualistic cosmic theory of the Yang and the Yin. According to this theory, Yang is a male principle, active and light, and it is represented by the heavens. Yin, on the other hand, is a female principle, which is passive, dark, and is represented by the earth.

The Chinese believe, that the human body, like matter is generally made up of five elements—wood, fire, earth, metal and water—and that each of these elements is associated with the five planets—the five conditions of the atmosphere, the five colours, the five stones, etc. Health, character and the success of all political and private ventures are pre-determined by the preponderance, at the time, of the Yang or the Yin. In the human body their proportions can be controlled, and this is the great objective of ancient Chinese medicine.

The Chinese are very ingenious and are highly remarkable in their medical therapeutics. Moxibustion which was introduced and practiced, consists in making a small, moistened cone of powdered leaves of mugwort or worm wood (Artemesia Sp.), applying it to the skin, igniting it and then crushing it into the blister so formed. The moistened cone of powdered leaves is known as the moxa, and other leaves and natural materials are used for preparing it, and for the treatment of skin diseases. But by far the most ingenious of the Chinese techniques is Acupuncture. This consists of insertion into the skin and underlying tissues of a hot or cold metal needle. The insertion is directed towards a particular organ or organs to insensitise the patient who can then undergo surgical operation without any attendant pain. The technique is still in use today despite the influence of modern medical science!

In Egypt, the early traditional doctors relied on herbs and extractives from plants for the treatment of diseases. Copper salts, castor oil inhalations, and gargles featured prominently in their prescriptions, as well as secretions and parts of animals. In addition, copious use was made of supernatural means, particularly, charms, and incantations. Medical practice was closely related to religion, and divination, as well as interpretation of dreams and astromonical happenings were made use of in treating the sick.

Traditional medical practice in Greece, the Middle East, and far Eastern countries, was therefore a combination of the use of supernatural powers in consonance with the religious beliefs and culture of the people, and of herbal remedies. As I mentioned earlier on, this practice still persists in spite of the dawn of civilisation, and the influence of western culture and modern medical science.

Traditional medicine was practised and is still practised, in developed countries and indeed the early traditional doctors came from Greece, Egypt, India and China. Even today we do have herbal clinics in countries like Britain, America, and in China, traditional doctors work in collaboration with modern doctors in the treatment of the sick.

Traditional doctors in Nigeria employ virtually the same methods used by traditional doctors in other lands, like Greece, the Middle East and far Eastern countries. These methods are a combination of the use of herbal remedies and of supernatural powers in consonance with the religious beliefs and culture of the people. There are various categories of traditional doctors in Nigeria. We have the curative doctors, who prescribe herbal remedies for diseases and ailments. These are known as the "Adahunse." Then there is the 'Babalawo' who consults his Ifa Oracle before prescribing necessary treatment. Other traditional doctors include the 'Oloya'—these are the worshippers of the River Niger; the worshippers of 'Sango' (Thunder called the 'Onisango'); the worshippers of Oshun River, known as the 'Oloshun'; the worshippers of 'Obatala'; known as the 'Olobatala'. All these in their own way diagnose ailments of patients and prescribe appropriate treatment within the context of their practice and beliefs.

Included in the category of traditional doctors are the various sects of prophets and prophetesses of different religious groups who are doing marvellous work in the cure and treatment of the sick. These category of doctors attract a large number of followers and adherents and their popularity is ever on the increase because of the wonderful nature of their work and achievement. They are rightfully classified as traditional doctors in that the essence of their practice is based on the tradition of ancient religious teachers and leaders (Chief of whom is Jesus Christ) and whose doctrine and teaching are being proclaimed and propagated. All these categories of traditional doctors acknowledge the existence of God and acclaim Him as the ominipotent and the ominiscient of their own existence and well being. The media which some of them use in their practice are no more than access routes through which they believe they can commune with God and get Him to do for them all that they ask of Him.

There is not much record about the early traditional doctors and their work in Nigeria, because these people could neither read nor write. What was known of them was what their associates, who are mainly the immediate members of their family learnt from them and passed on from one generation to the other. There is however a well known traditional doctor, by name Dr. J.O. Odumosu who was perhaps the most renowned and reputable doctor of his time. This man was not a qualified medical practitioner according to western standards. Nevertheless he was a highly remarkable man, whose skill in native medicine, and the free treatment and medical attention he gave to his people, earned for him the title "doctor."

Dr. Odumosu was literate and he made use of this in reducing his medical therapeutics into writing, using his native language "Yoruba." This book he published in many forms and sold at reasonable prices to the people. The two principal publications are "Iwe Egbogi"—(A book of Pharmacopaeia) and "Iwe Iwosan"—(A book of Healing Methods). These books proved very invaluable to the community, especially to the Yoruba speaking people. These publications however brought Dr. Odumosu into conflict with his fellow herbalists, who expressed great resentment and concern at the books, because they felt that Dr. Odumosu divulged the secrets of their trade by making it possible for everybody to know how to treat diseases, through the pages of books. This, according to them, meant that the herbalist would lose their patients, and so they the herbalists, would be thrown out of their jobs! As a result of this, reprint editions of the books were forbidden, and the circulation was thus curtailed.

Traditional doctors of different races and in different countries of the world did good pioneering work in the field of curative and preventive medicine. These doctors came mainly from Greece, Egypt, India and China, and of course from Africa and from Nigeria. The non-Africans were known as traditional doctors, and nothing in their practice was considered unusual and derogatory. But the African doctors constituted the native doctors—the word "native" connoting inferiority and all that is despicable. These doctors are the "jujumen" and the witch doctors who must not be allowed to exist much less thrive, according to the philosophy of our former colonial masters and christian missionaries. Despite this campaign of hate, the native doctors are very much with us and we prefer to address them as traditional doctors.

Let us now examine in some detail the peculiar features of the various types of traditional medical practice in Nigeria. The prescriptions of traditional doctors can be classified into three categories: (i) that which is made up of plant parts (ii) that which is a combination of plant parts and parts of animals or animal secretions (iii) that which is made up of plant parts, and/or parts of animals in combination with certain incantations which must be recited a given number of times and at stated hours of the day or night before, or with, or after the application of the remedial mixture. All these types of prescriptions are used for either curative or preventive treatment and with remarkable efficacy.

The late Dr. Odumosu aptly typified the traditional doctor, of his day. In his book on medical therapeutics he outlined in very clear terms, the preconditions which must be satisfied before effective treatment of the patient could be achieved. He made it clear that before any treatment was prescribed it must be ascertained that the patient did not suffer from constipation, and if he did, this must be corrected. He then went on to stress the importance of the life history of the patient and that of his immediate parents and family, as an important ingredient to correct diagnosis of the ailment.

Some of the questions usually asked the patient are as follows: (i) Do you know of any hereditary disease within your family? (ii) If so do you think your present complaint is hereditary? (iii) How long have you been suffering from this illness? (iv) Do you know the common local name for the disease? (v) Do you sleep well? (vi) Are your bowels free? (vii) What is the colour of your urine? and so on. After carefully considering the answers given by the patient, followed by a careful physical examination, a prescription was then given, which consisted mainly of herbs and various plant parts.

The Ifa priest, is a traditional doctor who relies on divination and on herbs for his practice. When a patient goes to the Ifa priest he is asked to say his complaint quietly and inaudibly to a piece of coin, which he then hands over to the priest. The priest then places the coin besides his 'Ifa oracle,' which he tosses up and down before laying it flat on the floor. He now 'reads' the oracle and proceeds to tell the patient the complaint which the patient had earlier on whispered to the piece of coin, inaudibly to the priest. The priest then goes on to read the horoscope of the patient and gives in detail the nature of his problems and difficulties from which he diagnoses the ailment.

Before prescribing a treatment, the priest usually recites some traditional historical poetry which is a narration of problems and misfortunes—similar to those of his patient— experienced by certain mystical and legendary figures, and the solutions and preventive measures which were then applied. He would then prescribe the appropriate treatment giving details of the application, and the incantation which must be recited by the patient, on, or before, or after application of the medicine. This prescription usually consists essentially of plant and/or animal parts.

In addition. where necessary, some sacrificial preparation —which invariably includes palm oil and other ingredients mainly of animal origin—is prescribed, and this has to be placed at a particular street or road junction, and at a specified time of night. This sacrificial preparation, must be carried in a special type of container and the carrier must not talk to anyone from the time it is carried and deposited, nor must he look back after depositing same till he reached the house from where he originally set out. The sacrificial preparation is meant to appease the evil spirits, and in order to be effective, none of the injunctions outlined above must be violated.

The Ifa priest is in the same category of traditional doctors as the chiefs of the various cults I mentioned earlier on. These cults have their own idols whom they worship and propitiate with sacrifices peculiar to, and characteristic of, the cult. The various cults direct their request to the idols who in turn furnish answers and solutions to the problems posed by the priest on behalf of the patient. In addition appropriate prescriptions are given, which usually consist of herbal and/or animal ingredients. There might or might not be some incantation to be recited with the application of the medicine, depending on the nature of the illness or the problem.

Surgical treatment is also given by the Nigerian traditional doctors. The treatment may be ordinary incissions of the affected part followed by application of powdered herbs. It may be cupping and blood-letting, or the removal of an obstruction by excission. In both cases the amputated part is washed with aqueous extract of herbs; and a medication of some plant part is applied either as a powder or in the form of an ointment consisting of an emulsion of oil or grease and powdered plant part.

Various other types of surgery, including orthopaedic surgery are practised by the traditional doctors. It is an open and well-known secret that traditional surgeons in this country are greater adepts at circumcision of males, than the modern surgeons. The traditional surgeon performs this operation of circumcision with a very sharp scalpel and the exposed crown of the male organ is bathed with the secretion of a snail—a very cold fluid which soothes the pain and stops the bleeding—after which the child is tied on to the back of the mother. The wound is then dressed with olive oil, and this dressing is repeated as often as necessary until the wound is completely healed.

There is another class of traditional doctors whose practice is based on religious beliefs and faith in the efficacy of prayers. Religious books like the christian Bible is full of stories of healing of the sick by prayers and faith. Indeed King Arthur was right when he said to Sir Bedevere: "More things are wrought by prayers than this world dreams of." The miraculous feeding of the 5,000 with only two fishes and five loaves of bread; the turning of water into wine at the marriage in Gaililee; the sudden appearance of the ram to Abraham when he was about to slaughter his only son as sacrificial offering in fulfilment of his solemn promises to God; the safety of Daniel in the den of lions; and the raising of Lazarus from the dead and restoration to life—all these are accounts which illustrate very vividly the power of faith and the efficacy of prayers.

It is against this background and the teachings of the acclaimed Leaders of religious faith that the traditional doctors who are followers of these leaders profess the same religion of faith and prayers and employ these in their ministry to the sick. The followers of Jesus Christ make use of the christian bible, whilst those of Mohammed make use of the Khoran. Both groups have very large following in this country, and are widely acclaimed.

Many people in this country are fully aware of the potentialities of these faith healers and can bear full testimony to the efficacy of their prayerful prescriptions. These faith healers are both curative and preventive. Preventive in that they foretell the future and future events with remarkable accuracy; and if these are perilous, they immediately warn the patient and then prescribe the preventive measures which largely consist of prayers and fasting, on behalf of the patient. In addition the patient is asked to adhere very rigidly to any injunction given by the healer, in order to avert the imminent danger.

The faith healers are curative in that they can heal patients also by prayers and fasting; and many patients who suffer from what has been regarded as incurable diseases have been effectively cured by these faith healers. Lunatics have been made sane; women have become mothers; and many miraculous feats have been achieved by these faith healers, for in the words of the Bible, which is the bed-rock of their practice—"all things are possible with God"—but only to those that believe and have implicit faith in the power of the Almighty. These faith healers can be classified as spiritualists, for they commune with the spirit through prayer and fasting, using the Bible or the Khoran as their only tool.

Traditional medicine and medical therapeutics are very diverse and comprehensive in nature and in their application. They cover all facets of life and have universal application. Peoples, the world over, enjoy the benefits of traditional medicine, and there are many who adhere strictly and rigidly to its use, and would never attend modern hospitals when they are ill. Such is the faith and confidence that people have in traditional medicine, that here in Nigeria, the clinics of the herbalists are always flooded, and the faith healers are continually besieged by people of all walks of life, with their complaints, in sure hope and belief that their health will be fully restored and their individual problems solved.

TRADITIONAL HEALING
AND THE MEDICAL/PSYCHIATRIC MAFIA

An Exclusive Interview with T. A. Lambo, M.D.
Deputy Director-General, World Health Organization, Geneva
By Philip Singer, Ph.D.

PS: *This is the World Health Organization. I'm in the office of Dr. Thomas A. Lambo in Geneva, and we will be discussing the World Health Organization and Dr. Lambo's view of traditional healing. Dr. Lambo is a Nigerian psychiatrist who was trained at Maudsley Psychiatric Institute in London between 1951 and 1954. He is presently the Deputy Director General of the World Health Organization; and, incidentally, as an American, it's probably worth noting that, as a black man he occupies the highest position in any international organization. But his reputation is not due to the fact that he is a black man occupying a significant position in an international organization. His reputation comes from the fact that he is an outstanding psychiatrist who was one of the very first, perhaps the first psychiatrist with impeccable credentials, coming from Maudsley, to try to integrate traditional methods of psychotherapeutic healing, psychiatric healing, with more orthodox Western psychiatric ways, including electric shock, drug therapy and various forms of psychotherapy. This was in the village of Aro in Abeokuta in Nigeria, primarily Yoruba country, where he worked with the chiefs, with the people, in setting up an institution which was totally unlike Dr. Schweitzer's Lamborene institution, which was remarkable as a noblesse oblige institution of the "Great White Father" serving Jesus and thereby serving the people. Dr. Lambo's institution at Aro was notable because it was a black scientist, a black psychiatrist, working with his own people within their own framework, not serving anybody except the cause of science and the cause of helping his own sick people.*

Now, Dr. Lambo, you are now Deputy Director General of World Health Organization. I wonder whether, since you have now occupied this basically very sensitive position, because all high bureaucratic positions are sensitive, whether you would now again think of starting a traditional healing center, with all the medical controversy that surrounds it.

TAL: Well, I think, I think I would consider starting some measure of traditional healing center, or some measure of traditional healing modalities, in different parts of the developing countries, not only in Africa, because it has become more and more obvious that the western approach to human health is not entirely acceptable to many people in other cultures.

PS: *When you say 'western approach,' as a Westerner, I understand that to mean primarily using drugs or tablets and electric shock and various other purely physiological and organic means to relieve disturbances. Is that what you mean by the 'western approach'?*

TAL: You're quite right. But at the same time, too, I also mean hospitalisation or institutionalisation. I feel that the Western approach tends to emphasise (1) disease entities; (2) the use of drugs and physiological mechanisms to look at man, whereas in other cultures we feel that there should be a hybrid situation.

PS: *There should be a hybrid situation?*

TAL: Yes. In other words, there should be a measure where we can probably use Western approaches in certain contexts, and at the same time within an overall local, cultural, socio-cultural approach.

PS: *But there's always the problem everywhere, whether it's with the traditional healer or whether it's with the physician, of who is responsible and who is in charge of the patient. Now who would you say would be in charge of the patient—the traditional healer or the western psychiatrist?*

TAL: I would be tempted to say the traditional healers, because here I am thinking in terms of the overall, the holistic approach, the totality of man. Rather than looking at him as a schizophrenic, we look at him as a person suffering from some disease entities.

PS: *Would it be fair to say—in speaking of the so-called schizophrenias and in speaking of the other functional illnesses by which we mean that there is no clearly discernible organic disorder—would it be fair to say instead of talking about them in terms of "disease entities," that they really represent problems in living, given our present state of knowledge?*

TAL: You're perfectly right. They represent certain disorganisation in human relationships, in the social context, disorganisation in the family context and so on. They represent what I call a disjunction in communication.

PS: *How would one go about working with traditional healers? We know that the governments of developing countries or emerging countries—countries that were formally called underdeveloped, but now go by these other names—we know that those countries have a great deal of pride in terms of trying to provide the best that they possibly can for their people, and that there's a strong feeling that the "best" means western psychiatric methods and they would tend probably not to want to use the backward, traditional, illiterate healers of their own culture.*

TAL: I think the opinions are changing gradually. In fact, I would say that a year ago, what you said now, was valid. Today, most of the developing countries, most of the leaders, the ministers of health, the policy makers, the politicans—are becoming much more sensitive to make things become much more local.

PS: *But what happened between a year ago and today? Change takes place very slowly; and for a year for a change like that to take place is phenomenal.*

TAL: It is actually, but what has been happening is that W.H.O. has become much more aggressive, much more active in this particular area. We have been more or less brainwashing the developing countries to say: "Look, you are despised because you're imitators. You must be able to use your own initiative; you must be able to be innovative. Go back to what you know, and begin to refine it."

PS: *Can you give some examples of some countries that are actively trying to use their own traditional cultures?*

TAL: Yes. For example, I've got a letter from the Minister of Health of India who's a Cambridge-trained person, and truly a sensitive, intelligent man and very powerful, who wrote to me and who saw me recently. He said that they would like to start something in India, and I do believe they've started to merge the western approach with the local approach. In fact, the local psychotherapeutic, traditional ways are being refined. In Kenya they've now started to look into this. W.H.O. is sending a paper to the Executive Board for the first time on traditional medicine. Nigeria has now decreed that measures should be taken to give license and so on and so forth. Well, these are innovative ideas. These are the signs of recognition that something has to be done.

PS: *Let's go back to the question I raised earlier. Is it possible to have a team approach between the western psychiatrically oriented physician, and the healer coming from his own culture? Again, who would be responsible for the patient on the team?*

TAL: I think it all depends. For example, when I was practicing in Nigeria, in Aro, we had a team approach and in certain areas or certain circumstances, I made the traditional healer in charge of the patient. In other instances, I was in charge and he was my collaborator. In fact, there was no such thing as a permanent head. We rotated. It depends on the context. It depends on whether the patient comes from the rural area and could not understand the modern psychiatrist and would like, for example, to have sacrifices done, have his dream interpreted and so on. It all depends.

PS: *Well, Dr. Lambo, this is not meant as criticism. In fact, it's a compliment. The fact is that you were able to achieve those things in Aro because of your own personality and because of your own awareness of the traditional culture. Now, I understand from my own recent visit to Nigeria that the team approach, the integrated approach that you pioneered so successfully for so many years in Aro has fallen by the wayside, because there is the conflict between the traditional healer and the western-trained psychiatrist. So does it then become a question of the particular empathy of a man like you, or is the approach that you recommend transferrable in terms of policy?*

TAL: I think that the approach which I recommend is transferrable in terms of policy. But in terms of implementation, it depends on the—I wouldn't use the word 'quality' of the man—it depends on the aggressivity of the man, his political status, because it was only a few days ago I was saying that psychiatry seems to be waning a little in strength. in Africa, whereas when I was there, I know all the politicians, I was able to participate in getting them better when they were ill. So psychiatry had a tremendous life, boost, and at the same time I was able to push it. Since I left, I think my younger boys have not had all the luck, and I feel that this has probably made things a little bit . . . .

PS: *I'd like to come back to something you just said about psychiatry waning. We said earlier that psychiatric disorders can be divided into functional, that is to say, of no organic basis, and organic, and the experience of psychiatrists and physicians all over the world is that between 60% and 80%, conservatively speaking, of the patients who come to their offices, who come to their clinics, are not suffering from any discernible organic disorder. Therefore, the question I want to ask is, is it necessary perhaps to take the whole functional area of so-called disorders away from the medical practitioner and put it back into the social worker, the Ph.D., the religious-healer, the community, in order to make the kind of progress in dealing with these disorders or problems of living, which are very real. Must it be removed from medicine?*

TAL: My own strong view would be that it should be in fact removed from traditional western medicine. When you feel, when you know in fact today that about 70% to 80% of those who are consulting, the physicians, whether as a surgeon, or optician or a pediatrician, that most of these people suffer from functional disorders of some sort because of the rapid change and the social-economic change, and so on, in different parts of the world—I feel that some of these other people who tackle the problems much better, much more effectively and less costly should be used to replace psychiatry. I think the cost is extremely important.

PS: *This sounds very revolutionary, but I would like to remind the listener that it is not revolutionary at all. Freud himself, the father of modern western psychiatry, recommended, and wished that the time would come when psychiatry would not belong to the physician. So although it may sound that what you said is very revolutionary it really goes back to the founder of psychiatry. But let us come back to a very real problem in the same area. Psychiatrists, after all, are just like chiefs, obeahmen, hunguns, voodo healers, kali mai healers, and the whole variety of curanderos and other indigenous healers. That is to say, they themselves have a vested interest in the patients that come to them and they don't want to give up power, money and responsibility. Do you see any fight between the traditional healers and the western psychiatrists?*

TAL: I think there will be a good deal of fight between the traditional healers and the western-trained psychiatrists. There won't be a great deal of difficulty in the developing countries because it is just emerging, and we could more or less combine the two and syncretise it, and emerge with a completely new approach or modality. In the old countries there would be a tremendous fight because actually I would not even go as far as to say that they have vested interests in terms of responsibility. I would say that they have vested interests in terms of money. What I have seen in North America alone really nauseates me. There are many times when I am in New York or in Washington and people say, "What do you do?" and I try to deny that I am a psychiatrist.

PS: *Well, explain a bit further as to why it nauseates you.*

TAL: Most of the people who go into psychiatry in North America today are going into it because of the tremendous benefit. Secondly, there is a great deal of what I call completely an unscientific approach, in that patients are being maintained far too long, almost all their life, to become entirely dependent, brainwashed. And I feel that this is not the approach.

PS: *Isn't there also another problem? You mentioned North America, being nauseated by the way things are going on there. I think that's strong and courageous judgment on your part. I've just come from England, specifically from the mental institution in Inverness, Scotland which is a 900-bed mental hospital and the center where all of the patients from the Outer Hebrides are sent. Patients come suffering mainly from problems of alcoholism and the depression that accompanies alcoholism. In my discussion with the psychiatrists*

247

and other personnel there, I asked them what type of treatment they provided for the patients. They said that they provide primarily electric shock, tranquillizers and a drying-out period. I asked, does it make any difference what the particular diagnosis is of the patient, in terms of the treatment? They said no. So if diagnosis, which is the sine qua non of medicine, is so totally unimportant in psychiatry, where the treatment is the same regardless, then what's the purpose of psychiatry anyway except to make money for those who are practicing?

TAL: You're quite right. As I see things in Europe and North America especially, it is less time-consuming to use tranquillizers, it is less time-consuming to use electric shock, whereas to go into a person's problems, social problems, human problems, psychodynamically, will take you a lot of time. And this, in fact, is one of the tremendous human qualities of the traditional healers. That they can listen, they really have tremendous interest, emotional empathy and relationship. And at the same time, too, it is not one-to-one type of psychotherapy: it is, in fact, a group type of psychotherapy.

PS: *Dr. Lambo, you have been outstandingly frank. I'm surprised. I never expected the Director—I promoted you,— the Deputy Director General would be as frank in his opinions about a subject which is usually glossed over with all kinds of bureaucratic doubletalk. And speaking of bureaucratic doubletalk, I have in front of me a report from the World Health Organization, Geneva, 1975, Technical Report Series No. 564 titled: "The Organization of Mental Health Services in Developing Countries." I'm afraid that the comments you have just made would never appear in this report. How can you—and I wish, I'd like to change our subject for a moment, if I may—how can you, who have such strong opinions, such courageous opinions, such provocative opinions based on expertise—how can you reconcile the bland, I would even say, nauseating, type of recommendations that come out of such a consensus report, which doesn't contain among its board of experts any traditional healers, and is dominated by the psychiatric profession. Don't you develop some kind of frustration when these kinds of reports emerge out of your Organization?*

TAL: No, I don't think so. I think the idea, at the present

moment, is that we are feeling much better, much easier about things of this nature. In the past, of course, one would worry a great deal, but we know that things are changing very rapidly. If you look at the list of participants you'll find that most, if not all, were from Western countries with probably a few individuals from the developing countries. And those people were even hand-picked, so that there won't be any sort of what I would call unorthodox views being expressed.

PS: *Exactly.*

TAL: Yes, but since then, of course, things are moving very rapidly.

PS: *You mean from 1975 . . .*

TAL: Since . . .

PS: *to 1975. Things are moving rapidly?*

TAL: You're quite right. Things are moving rapidly. So much so that only yesterday I signed the paper of the traditional healing—the Executive Board paper, which, if you see, you'd be absolutely staggered.

PS: *Can you tell us a little bit about this?*

TAL: Yes, we're now proposing to the Executive Board which will go to the Assembly that there should be some measure of integration of traditional healing. That each Member State should examine critically all the modalities in their culture, at their disposal, and that at the same time be able to salvage as much as possible to syncretize and integrate this. And this is completely unusual. In fact, for the time we are laying ourselves wide open.

PS: *In fact, I'd say it's a manifesto; it's a revolutionary manifesto.*

TAL: Absolutely revolutionary. And there is going to be a great deal of resistance, antagonisms; there'll be the mafia of the world . . .

PS: *The mafia of the world—I like that. Who'd you describe as the mafia of the world?*

TAL: I wouldn't like to mention them. I'm sure . . . ha, ha, ha . . .

PS: *Alright, alright. Well, for the benefit of the listeners who may not be as knowledgeable as to the medical mafia of the world. I won't identify them per se. I would simply say that they represent the dominant medical organizations in*

that they represent the dominant medical organizations in whatever country where the medical profession happens to be dominant. I suppose though as an American, I'd have no hesitation in saying that in America it represents the American Psychiatric Association and the American Medical Association, but let's come back to this revolutionary document that we have just been talking about. Is it possible that the World Health Organization may one day convene a World Health Organization Expert Committee on Mental Health which would include traditional healers—traditional healers who are illiterate but very literate in terms of their culture—traditional healers who cannot speak the language of the round tables or the oval tables of Geneva but who can speak beautifully in terms of the patois, the dialect of their own culture? Is it possible that we may see a conference of traditional healers comprising an Expert Committee of World Health Organization?

TAL: Professor Singer, I think that you are more or less reading my thoughts. In fact, we are hoping that if the document goes through the Assembly, the Executive Board, and is well accepted, that by March, 1976 we'll have what I call a Consultation Group. I wouldn't call them an Expert Committee, but a Consultation Group of people whom I think will be the really Western oriented—who will passionately defend the historical and their own stand—as well as people from Africa, Asia and Latin America who are fairly articulate, who know exactly what they are doing and yet not trained in the Western. It will be the first time in the history of the Organization to have such a Consultation Group.

PS: *Exactly. In that connection, realistically speaking—realistically because you are the Deputy Director General of the World Health Organization: you understand the medical mafia of the world as well as the medical mafia of the World Health Organization—realistically speaking, do you think that such a resolution—such a document as you have spoken about just now—can possibly be approved by the World Health Organization?*

TAL: Well, I think it will be approved by the World Health Organization Assembly because as you know yourself that in the assembly of most of the agencies and the Assembly of the U.N., there is a great voice of the developing countries. I wouldn't say that they are dominated by the developing countries, but for the first time in the history of the United Nations, the people, the views of the people of the developing countries, are now being heard, and their votes are very important indeed.

PS: *Well, that's true, but still, I know myself from having been in many of the developing countries, that although there are cabinet ministers, although there are politicians, although there are leaders in the government who go to the traditional healers themselves, they do so quietly, sub rosa, at midnight when people will not recognize their cars or the licenses on their cars or who they are, and I'm not sure that such people in developing countries, representing their own countries, would be willing to say I who am a MD or PhD from Edinburgh or from the university in the United States, I go to a traditional healer, because then they would be laid open to charges of magic, superstition, supernaturalism. Do you think they would be prepared to passionately espouse the cause of traditional healing?*

TAL: I think they would, if only purely on political grounds. I think they would if purely on the grounds of pride. I use the word 'political' grounds to emphasize the new philosophy of self reliance of the developing countries. They really feel proud that they would like to scientifically explore the things which they have discarded. For example, after Nigerian independence, most of us went back to native gowns and agbadas and so on. Before that I was trained by the Baptists. I was told to discard all the images as savage, uncivilized, and so on and so forth. Even our dances were sensual and everything was unthinkable. But a rear guard action was fought immediately after independence, and I feel that the same type of attitude, mood, is being expressed now by politicians.

PS: *Again, however, I think it is important to emphasize that while we are talking in this vein, it is only because most psychiatric disorder is of a functional nature which is responsive to the symbolic system which is responsive to the cultural assumptions of the particular culture. This is basically what we are talking about. We are not talking about 'organic' disorders; we are talking about 'functional' disorders, which I suppose another word for it could be 'cultural' disorders.*

TAL: Well, I think you are quite right, but I would also like to emphasize that in many countries—non-Western countries—even in organic states there is what we call 'functional overlay.' And if a person feels much more relaxed and really at peace, the body functions—the physiological functions—will be able to recover so that there is also a large area of the organic which has a mixture with the functional.

PS: *Can you tell us when will the World Health Organization special meeting of the General Assembly be held which will consider this resolution?*

TAL: The paper—the document—is going to the Executive Board in January, 1976 and then, if all goes well, it will be recommended by the Executive Board to the Assembly in May, 1976. And we are hoping that by the end of the year, next year, there will be tremendous exposure.

PS: *Well, I don't think there's any doubt that this particular approach—this particular document—is as great a revolution in psychiatry as was the freeing of the patients from their chains by Pinel in the nineteenth century in France. And it's been really a remarkable pleasure to hear a bureaucrat, because you are a bureaucrat, speak as straight and frankly as you have. I wish you every success in this revolution that you are trying to create in the World Health Organization. Thank you very much.*

November 15, 1975

NKPORA AGREEMENT

Philip Singer

In December 1973, I participated in the International Symposium* on "Traditional Medical Therapy—A Critical Appraisal," held at the University of Lagos, and sponsored by the University, the Lagos State Government Ministry of Health and the Nigeria Association of Medical Herbalists.

. It seems to me that the major problem facing the traditional healers is not the opposition to them by modern medicine practitioners, who they overwhelmingly outnumber, but their own internal factional splits over questions of secrecy, experimentation, organization, leadership. It is clear that as far as "clientele" is concerned, there is no shortage of patients for the traditional indigenous physicians, wherever they are, Africa, Asia, or the U.S.A. Therefore, the problem is not cooperation with the modern physicians, but competition among themselves. The disputes here cannot be dignified as searches for the best, or affirmation of cultural identity, it is simply a struggle for power. The disputants are not colonialists and anti-colonialists. They are all traditionalists.

There is more indication, however, that among the traditionalists, there are those who would like to synthesize the best from the traditional and the modern. This movement is summed up in the Nkpora Agreement, which follows here. If the Nkpora Agreement is realized, then it will be possible to professionalize the traditional healing methods with research, experimentation, indigenous pharmacopeias, case studies, hospitals, and eventual accreditation systems. At this time, with the exception of the accrediting systems that exist in modern medicine and its practitioners, there is no way to determine who is a charlatan and who is a bona-fide traditional healer. Any one may hang out his shingle and attach to it any and all degrees, including that of "Ph.D. in Miracles." (sic).

*Proceedings of the International Symposium on "Traditional Medical Therapy—A Critical Appraisal," Dec. 10-16, 1973. Mimeo.

Although traditional healers I have talked to, including Chief Lambo, point to the Communist Chinese use of indigenous healers and the "barefoot doctors," they are neither aware, nor interested in knowing that the Chinese "barefoot doctors" are part of a massive, state-controlled system of government medicine and very much at the control of the central government, and with a philosophy basically in opposition to traditional healing. This is something the traditional healers in Nigeria definitely do not want. It also seems absolutely clear that if a dual system of traditional medicine and modern medicine is established in Nigeria with government support, inevitably there would be more investment, more resources, more facilities given to the modern institutions than to the traditional systems. This would be so if for no other reason than that the traditional systems are not technology-generating systems oriented around scientific methods of diagnosis, surgery, medication, etc., but depend entirely, at this point, on symbolic reinforcement. The only area in which they could generate technology and resources would be in the materia medica area, and here there is still so much private, secret entrepreneurship, that it seems an unlikely eventuality in the near future. I need to add, however, that this is not true of the adherents of the Nkpora Agreement who welcome cooperation with the modernists. Here, however, the problem seems to be that the western oriented physicians and institutions do not apparently feel that the indigenous pharmacopeia is worthy of their investment.

Implementation of the Nkpora Agreement would be a significant step forward in a meaningful relationship between traditional and modern medicine.

NOTES ON CONTRIBUTORS

A. Akisanya, Ph.D. is Fellow of the Royal Institute of Chemistry, London, and Dean, Faculty of Science, University of Lagos, Nigeria.

Enrique Araneta, Jr. is Associate Professor of Psychiatry at the University of Florida, College of Medicine and Assistant Chief, Psychiatric Service at the V.A. Hospital, Gainesville, Florida. He is a diplomate in Psychiatry, American Board of Neurology and Psychiatry. He was born in the Philippines on May 4, 1925, graduated from Medical School in 1948 from the University of the Philippines, College of Medicine. Between 1948-1962, he was an instructor in Human Anatomy and Embryology, College of Medicine, University of the Philippines and between 1952-1956, was Assistant Professor of Anatomy and Neuroanatomy, Institute of Medicine, Far Eastern University.

While undergoing post-graduate training in Neurology, Albany Medical College, he taught post-graduate Neuro-anatomy. He was Assistant Professor and consultant in Neuroanatomy. He was Assistant Professor and consultant in Neurology at the Far Eastern University and Institute of Medicine, 1961-1962. He was head of Mental Health Services and Medical Superintendent of Fort Canje Hospital, British Guiana, South America. Between 1966 and 1969 he was Unit Chief, Psychiatric Service, VA Hospital, Albany, New York and between 1970 and 1973, was Chief of Neurology and Psychiatry Service, V.A. Center, Hampton, Virginia. His interests and publications range from cultural psychiatry to neurology.

A. B. Dawkins, Jr. is Former Health Worker, Career Escalation and Training Program, Lincoln Community Mental Health Center, Bronx, New York.

Ruth G. Dawkins is Former Director, Career Escalation and Training Prgoram, Lincoln Community Mental Health

Center, Bronx, New York.

In a letter to Dr. Philip Singer in 1971, at the time the paper on "indigenous Healing" was written for a Symposium the editor had organized for the Society for Applied Anthropology, the Dawkins wrote from the Bronx, New York:

> Although we have been to colleges and attended classes in speech, writing, psychiatry, etc., etc., all traditional and structural, they have all proven to be ineffective in dealing with our people. We have cast aside all this white computerized programming, and work through what is part of Third World People and that is "Vibrations."

Chief J. O. Lambo, President General of the Nigeria Association of Medical Herbalists, was born in 1915 at Abeokuta, Western State of Nigeria. He has been interested in herbalism since 1934 and he taught at high schools and the Baptist Academy School from 1940 to 1962. He has been a Chief since 1969. He is a member of many social, occult and religious societies and he is also an astrologer and a member of the Rusicrucian Fellowship. His senior brother, Professor T. A. Lambo, is presently Deputy Director General of the World Health Organization at Geneva.

John Langrod is a Research Psychologist, Albert Einstein College of Medicine, Yeshiva University, New York City.

F. M. Mburu, a native of Kenya, is on study leave from the University of Nairobi, Faculty of Medicine, Department of Community Medicine, where he has been a member of the staff since June, 1972. He obtained his B.A. in sociology in 1972 from Makerere University, Kampala, Uganda. A field survey and a thesis entitled "Traditional and Modern Medicine Among the Akamba Ethnic Group" written in 1973, gained him a M.A. from Makerere.

Since March, 1972 he has also been conducting research as part of a longitudinal study on medical, socioeconomic, cultural, demographic and geographical factors in child morbidity and mortality under the auspices of the Medical Research Center, Nairobi, Department of the Royal Tropical Institute, Amsterdam. Besides being interested in the utilization and organization of health services, he is currently a Doctoral student, Department of Health Care Administration, School of Pharmacy, University of Mississippi.

Simon D. Messing holds the Ph.D. in Anthropology from the University of Pennsylvania, 1957. Field work included ethnographic research in Ethiopia, 1953-1954, on a grant from the Ford Foundation, and 1961-1967 in Ethiopia as a U.S. Foreign Service Officer with USAID-Public Health. Teaching included the years 1956-1958 at Paine College, 1958-1960 at Hiram College, Ohio, 1960/1 and 1963/4 at the University of South Florida, and since 1968 at Southern Conn. State College, New Haven. In addition to the unpublished Ph.D. dissertation, "The Highland-Plateau Amhara of Ethiopia," 1957, Dr. Messing has published the paperback, *The Target of Health in Ethiopia*, MSS Information Corp, New York 1972; has edited the monograph, *Rural Health in Africa*, African Studies Center, East Lansing, Mich. 1972, and articles such as "Group Therapy and Social Status in the Zar Cult of Ethiopia" (in Opler, M.K.: *Culture and Mental Health*, Macmillan, 1959).

J. O. Mume, N.D., D.O., Ph.D., is the President of Jom Tradomedical Research Group, which is located in Agbarho, Via Warri, in the Midwestern State, Nigeria. The Group which claims to be the "only organization in Nigeria and Africa," has three objectives: a) to advocate and conduct research into Nigerian traditional medicine and all sciences associated with the healing or treatment of diseases by natural methods; b) to raise the status and protect the general interests of practitioners of traditional medicine; and c) to establish hospitals for traditional medicine and laboratories for the manufacture of herbal medicines.

K. O. K. Onyioha is Chief High Priest of the Gordian Religion of Nigeria.

Pedro Ruiz, M.D. is Associate Professor of Psychiatry and Director, Lincoln Community Mental Health Center,

Albert Einstein College of Medicine, Yeshiva University, New York City.

John H. Shepherd was born in Detroit, Michigan and received degrees in Economics and Law from the University of Michigan. He studied on a Fulbright Scholarship at the Law School of the University of Paris, France, and subsequently taught International Law, Constitutional Law and American Government at Wayne State University in Detroit. He is a partner in the law firm of Sommers, Schwartz, Silver, Schwartz, Tyler & Gordon, P.C. with offices in Detroit and Southfield. He serves as Consul in Michigan for the Republic of Ivory Coast.

Philip Singer received his Ph.D. in Anthropology from Syracuse University in 1961. He taught for six years at the Albany Medical Center Hospital and College in Albany, New York. For two years he was a member of the United Nations Secretariat, New York. He is currently Professor of Health-Medical Behavioral Sciences and Anthropology, Oakland University, Rochester, Michigan. He also is Adjunct Professor of Community Medicine, Michigan State University. He is a member of the Group for Medical Anthropology; the International Committee on Traditional Medical Therapy; and the President of the American branch of the Nigerian Medical Herbalist Association. He is also a consultant in Ethnopsychiatry to the Veterans Administration Hospital, Hampton, Virginia.

Loudell F. Snow holds the Ph.D. degree in Anthropology from the University of Arizona. She investigated the medical belief system in a predominantly black neighborhood in Tucson for her doctoral thesis. Since 1971 she has been Assistant Professor of Anthropology and Assistant Professor of Community Medicine at Michigan State University. She is involved in teaching medical students in both the College of Human Medicine and the College of Osteopathic Medicine. She is also the behavioral scientist member of a campus-based primary health care team. Her area of special interest is American folk medicine, in particular witchcraft beliefs and practices, the folklore of the female reproductive cycle, and unorthodox healers. She and her teenage son live in East Lansing, Michigan.

Joseph Westermeyer, M.D. is Associate Professor, Department of Psychiatry, University of Minnesota, Minneapolis, Minnesota.

Charles H. Williams was born in Southeast Michigan and attended the University of Michigan for his undergraduate study. He took his D.O. from the Kirksville College of Osteopathic Medicine in 1953. He interned at Mt. Clemens General from 1953-54. He has been in general practice in the Southeast Michigan area for 20 years. At present he is in a psychiatric residency at Clinton Valley Center for the mentally ill at Pontiac, Michigan, and associated with the School of Human Medicine at Michigan State University, Lansing, Michigan. Also for the past two years he has taken post graduate work in social anthropology at Oakland University in the department of History and Anthropology with concentration in the folk healing practices of Mexican-Americans. He has been a guest lecturer at Oakland University in the department of Behavioral Science on the psychological aspects of General Practice.